Cardiothoracic Handbook

Cardiothoracic Handbook
A pocket companion

A. Hedley Brown, MS, FRCS
Consultant Cardiothoracic Surgeon

Fernando Guzman M, MD, IGACS
Senior Registrar

Regional Cardiothoracic Centre,
Freeman Hospital,
Newcastle upon Tyne

Butterworths
London Boston Singapore Sydney Toronto Wellington

First published, 1988

© **Butterworth & Co. (Publishers) Ltd, 1988**

British Library Cataloguing in Publication Data

Hedley Brown, A.
  Cardiothoracic handbook.
  1. Man. Cardiovascular system. Surgery
  2. Man. Thorax. Surgery
  I. Title   II. Guzman M, Fernando
  617′.41

ISBN 0–407–01743–7

Library of Congress Cataloging-in-Publication Data

Hedley Brown, A.
  Cardiothoracic handbook.

  Bibliography: p.
  Includes index.
  1. Heart—Surgery—Handbooks, manuals, etc.
  2. Chest—Surgery—Handbooks, manuals, etc. 3. Heart—Diseases—Handbooks, manuals, etc. 4. Chest—Diseases—Handbooks, manuals, etc. I. Guzman M., Fernando.
  II. Title.
  RD598.H429   1988   617′.412   88–28527

ISBN 0–407–01743–7

Typeset by Latimer Trend & Company Ltd, Plymouth
Printed and bound in England by Hartnoll Ltd, Bodmin, Cornwall

Preface

Over the past 20 years the advances made in the field of cardiac and thoracic surgery have been amazingly rapid, making it impossible to cover every month's medical and surgical literature reading. Since the first conception of this handbook it has been our hope to help the current generation of trainees approach with confidence the diverse and acute problems of surgical cardiothoracic patients, especially those cases in whom quick decisions make the difference between life and death. Such confidence is particularly important when consultant support is not immediately available.

In the characteristically busy UK cardiothoracic unit, the trainees have very limited time for theory during the first months of training, and the amount of information is such that formulae, dosages and numbers are not easily recalled under stress. Therefore, this handbook is addressed to those members of the junior staff who are trying to build up their basic skills.

It is not for the erudite. Nevertheless, we have found it very rewarding that the booklet from which this manual has evolved is often consulted by our colleagues who give us feedback with new suggestions and constructive criticism.

Our thanks are extended to Butterworths, and particularly to Mr John Harrison, Senior Commissioning Editor, who encouraged us to jump from the local edition to a wider publication, and to D. Crawford, O.D.A. who did the drawings.

A. Hedley Brown
Fernando Guzman M

Contents

Section I.

Cardiac Medicine

The duties of a house doctor

The currency on the doctor's side of his contract with the public is the provision of medical care and the proper stewardship of knowledge, which implies the accumulation of existing medical facts, the discovery of unknown facts, and the imparting of this knowledge to colleagues. Both these aspects of a doctor's duty can well be fulfilled in a somewhat feudal system, in that the flow of responsibility can be upwards and the flow of knowledge and experience downwards. Resident staff must therefore consult their seniors, and keep them posted on day to day occurrences, as well as evoking instruction by questioning consultant policies rather than accepting them as dogma. The contribution of the man on the spot to practical matters of management can be great. Finally, to read around the clinical problem is as much part of one's duty in a training post as is the participation in the treatment of these problems. It may also contribute towards the postgraduate education of one's seniors.

The word 'house' or 'resident' is inseparable from the role of the most junior hospital doctor. In it lies the key to his invaluable place in the medical family, and the explanation for the rapidity with which medical maturity develops in this period of his career. He is present. By being so he is fulfilling the substance of his obligations. Commuting housemen, external interns or non-resident residents do not even fulfil the shadow of their obligations, even to themselves.

Duties in most institutions begin at 8 a.m. and most hospital charts, duty changes, etc. change at this hour. House staff should have an afternoon a week by arrangement for study, and at these times and at weekends and nights off there should be no work undone before he leaves, and his relieving doctor should be thoroughly conversant with the patients who become his responsibility. A formal handing-over procedure, preferably in the ward and not in the bar, must precede all departures. The ward staff and the telephone operators must be informed of the transfer of responsibility.

1

The documentation of medical data is educational, ensures that the data are actually obtained, forms the baseline for future medical encounters for a patient, provides proof that medical care and interest are of a sufficient standard and is the incentive to make them of that standard. This documentation is thus of highly medical significance and educational importance and is not a non-clinical chore but a vital duty of the houseman, by which not only he, but his firm, may be judged.

Much tiresome form-filling has been eliminated by the introduction of labels with all the patient's basic information on them, and by the recruitment of ward clerks. This does not absolve the clinician from the duty of basic civility to his behind-the-scenes colleagues in the form of an indication of why an investigation is requested, and supporting hard data if available. If an unusual request is made, a personal word with the pathologist or radiologist concerned is usually easy and vastly improves the quality of care and interest of all concerned. Attendance in the X-ray department is of great value to clinicians, radiologists and patients. Thus the investigation-requesting part of one's life can be a vital experience rather than tiresome pen-pushing.

Recruitment of nursing, theatre and intensive care staff is below requirements, usually because of human dissatisfaction with the tasks, usually rooted in a feeling of not being in the picture. As liaison man, the friendly houseman plays a crucial part. His labour of public relations, informing ward, theatre, intensive care staff, blood bank and clinical laboratories and X-ray departments of forthcoming work plans, and the likely course of events, or reasons for changes of routine, are thus of immense human importance and again should not be regarded as administrative chores.

Consultation with other specialists can be a stimulating part of the daily round if properly set up. All too often the poor chap gets a scribbled note reminiscent of the GP referral to Casualty Department – 'PUO, please C' – and turns up unannounced to find out the patient's whereabouts from an indifferent ward maid, makes his diagnosis and writes it in the notes where he has no guarantee it will ever be read. The houseman can ensure that his consultant and the visitor meet over the problem, have all the necessary data for their fruitful discussion, and do their discussing in circumstances where the educational value of it is not wasted, and the decisions can be promptly implemented to the satisfaction of all concerned.

The prescribing of medicines is the very ethos of doctoring, and while it must be done scrupulously (or its metric equivalent) it could never be dismissed as clerical work. Similarly, the discharge letter with a complete account of current treatment is both an important assurance of continuity of medical care and a shop window for the firm's reputation, together with the case summary whose promptness and lucidity are the basis for external evaluation of a medical unit.

The distribution of the case load should be clear. Thus several junior staff on a firm should demarcate their responsibilities clearly and never fail to fulfil them. Amorphous communal work-sharing should be shunned. When there are several consultants in a firm and several junior staff, every effort should be made to make 'cells' of small numbers in which the responsibility would not be unduly diluted. The houseman should document all admissions occurring during working hours under his consultant, whether they be from the waiting list, emergencies, or transfers. His substitute should attend to emergencies completely, and check that no immediate action is necessary in the other cases. Housemen should examine their own cases twice daily, and have a full and up-to-date knowledge of the cases on the closely related 'cells' of a unit, plus those patients under their care as an out-of-hours substitute.

Ward rounds should be done in the company of the head nurse of the ward, to ensure the immediate reception of recommendations for management; it is thus important that they should be timed for a convenient time for the constant attendance of the sister without other distractions. The worst choice of time for these events is a mealtime when the sister is presiding over the distribution of food and the patients are all away from their beds and charts, which are all piled up on the day room desk being neatly marked; at all costs, even that of a few extra minute's rest, doctors should ensure that they catch the sister, the charts and the patients at the ward bed, with procedures book, prescription sheets and ward clerk simultaneously on hand to execute decisions made. A daily round of this thoroughness, and an evening round of a quieter sort, are the minimum necessary. A round should always be done in preparation for the consultant's round.

When patients arrive in operating theatre the irreversible condition of starting the operation is imminent, and this is a most unsuitable time to discover omissions in the pre-operative work-up. The operation should have been explained to the patient and his/her consent to it obtained. A check list should have been followed by the houseman the night before, in anticipation of the arrival of the anaesthetist to write up the premedication.

Any alteration of a theatre list should be notified to the ward and the patient, the operating theatre, blood bank, any other investigation facilities involved such as frozen section department, pump and pressure technicians, recovery and intensive care ward, and anaesthetist. X-ray screening and medical electronics should be notified of changes in plans for pacemaker implantation.

In the operating theatre the junior staff should be delegated to tasks within their capability and of an ever increasing degree of complexity and skill, so that they feel constantly that they are making progress. Postoperatively the theatre book should be confirmed as having been correctly filled in, the operation form in the patient's record completed, the daily follow-up note of the patient should enumerate the procedures, and all specimens correctly labelled and sent for analysis with helpful details. The junior staff should view the final dressings and see the patients off the table and back to the ward, recovery ward or intensive care unit, and see that they are properly settled, supervised, ventilated, etc. there, and that immediate management is detailed to the staff receiving the patient.

Discharge of patients should be well anticipated, all concerned being notified in good time and transport and other arrangements completed in an unhurried manner. The discharge report must be sent at this time, the notes completed and sorted, and the Registrar thus furnished with all the data necessary for immediate completion of the case summary.

Death of a patient should be notified immediately to the consultant and the general practitioner and the discharge report sent forthwith. The Coroner's office should be notified if a death occurs other than from 'natural' causes. Permission for autopsy should be obtained and summary sent to the pathologist.

Outpatient's follow-up often falls to the lot of the junior staff, and is a worthwhile source of reassurance to them that their inpatient treatment was justified and fruitful. It is the basis of the clinical follow-up report and an important source of feedback to the firm of the success of its policies. The junior staff should not, therefore, feel these sessions to be a chore.

At all stages of a patient's progress through hospital, the house staff should take seriously their role as the liaison officer with the relatives. An official time should be set aside each day for an interview with the relatives of inpatients, and contact made whenever major changes in the patient's progress occur. Explanations of operations and other treatments should be made, and the statistical information of risks, benefits, etc., when available, should be detailed. Before admission the likely stay and course of events should be described to the family and at review they should not be left out of the picture. If the houseman does not feel he has all the necessary information, or that his words lack weight, he should ask his senior colleagues to talk to the relatives.

The Registrar's role

A Registrar's duties are of an executive nature as well as a technical medical one. Upon his coordinating skill depends the smooth flow of services offered to patients, and he must see them through all phases of the experience.

The provision and efficient turnover of beds for routine and emergency patients is the responsibility of the Registrar in consultation with the ward sister with, if available, the help of the ward clerk. The Registrar is the point of contact with the GP where the unit's reputation is at stake. He must therefore answer calls promptly, handing over his bleep when going into theatre to someone like the receptionist who can relay urgent calls for him. Referrals should be housed without a wait for confirmation that there is room and only when a second opinion rather than admission is requested should the Registrar 'vet' prospective admissions in Casualty Department before confirming admission.

While the patient is in the ward the Registrar should hasten progress by optimal coordination of investigation and treatment, and should ensure the accurate recording of clinical data by the houseman, and the prompt insertion of investigation results, which he should scrutinize frequently.

Tidy case notes make the Registrar's task of summarizing the patient's course easier and probably more prompt after the patient's discharge, at which time the Registrar should also ensure that the patient's treatment is noted, discharge prescription and doctor's letter were completed by the houseman. A Registrar is in training, and should always make independent assessment of patients, which should be recorded; he should fill the gaps in the houseman's work-up and request investigations not already ordered to support his opinions.

He should teach his juniors and arrange his movements so as to learn from his seniors and visiting specialists, and attend and participate in as many of the postgraduate educational events in his area as possible.

He should attend all operation lists unless specifically excused, and should not miss outpatients' sessions except for good reasons. Registrars should be doing research as well as learning their trade, and should read journals and hold journal club meetings in addition to accumulating basic textbook knowledge.

Discharge

The last impression of the patient of his hospital stay is probably the longest lasting and, with the immediate discharge letter and summary, is the shop window of the unit. Well timed, well prepared, thoughtful discharge with social as well as medical considerations in mind, round off the excellence of the management. District nurses and GPs will enjoy participating in such a train of events, and should be well primed to do so. Convalescent centres are precious commodities and will be more available to those units which show them consideration.

The patient should be given a letter with all his treatment and management plans to take with him. A copy of these should be written in the case notes (not a carbon stuffed into the mixture of bumph in the back of the folder).

A prompt and full summary of the case should be dispatched by the Registrar, and adequate follow-up arrangements confirmed.

Admission procedure

Generally the routine patients are clerked by the doctor on the ward to which he goes, and emergencies and transfers are clerked by the duty doctor immediately. Day cases should be seen, summarized and medicated by the doctor not in the operating theatre as soon as they arrive.

Pre-operative history and examination should be full from the general point of view, but should also specifically include, for all heart cases, the items listed below.

History

(1) *Raised left atrial pressure*: dyspnoea I to IV (grading of exercise limitation – the endpoint of the titration is the need to stop the activity because of the symptom: Grade I prevents athletic activities; IIa hurrying; IIb normal walking; III even slow walking is interrupted by the symptom; Grade IV the symptom disturbs rest). Also, paroxysmal nocturnal dyspnoea, orthopnoea and pulmonary oedema.

(2) *Increased bronchial venous pressure*: exercise cough, bronchitis, haemoptysis.

(3) *Right heart failure*: oedema, ascites, hepatic pain.

(4) *Arrhythmias*: slow, fast, irregular, extra, missed, or abnormal beats.

(5) *Angina*: not other chest pain syndrome. Grades I to IV – number of spontaneous attacks per month, provocation by emotion, cold or heavy meals.

(6) *Lowered cardiac output*: fatigue of true cardiac type, syncope, sudden death.

(7) *Emboli*: loss of use of limbs or speech, splenic pain, haematuria.

Also 'other health', past health, drug history, family history and social history.

Examination

(1) *General*: stigmata of cardiac-associated abnormalities of congenital (Marfan's, Down's, Holt Oram, moonface) or acquired (arcus senilis, xanthomata) type; stigmata of cardiac disease (cyanosis, clubbing, malar flush, cardiac cachexia) or of conse-

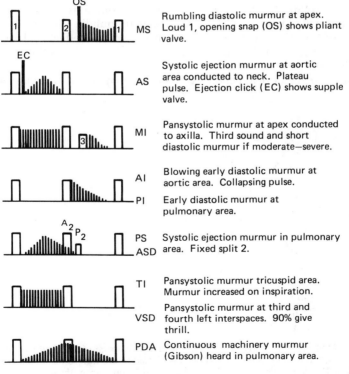

MS — Rumbling diastolic murmur at apex. Loud 1, opening snap (OS) shows pliant valve.

AS — Systolic ejection murmur at aortic area conducted to neck. Plateau pulse. Ejection click (EC) shows supple valve.

MI — Pansystolic murmur at apex conducted to axilla. Third sound and short diastolic murmur if moderate–severe.

AI — Blowing early diastolic murmur at aortic area. Collapsing pulse.

PI — Early diastolic murmur at pulmonary area.

PS — Systolic ejection murmur in pulmonary
ASD — area. Fixed split 2.

TI — Pansystolic murmur tricuspid area. Murmur increased on inspiration.

VSD — Pansystolic murmur at third and fourth left interspaces. 90% give thrill.

PDA — Continuous machinery murmur (Gibson) heard in pulmonary area.

Figure 1.1 Cardiac function: auscultation

quences or complications of cardiac disease (splinter haemorrhages and neuroembolic damage).

(2) *Pulse*: rate, rhythm, tension (and blood pressure), volume, wave and wall, peripheral pulses, radiofemoral timing, palpable collaterals.

(3) *Jugular venous pressure*: height, wave form.

(4) *Cardiac impulse*: position, left ventricular or right ventricular chamber or outflow tract hyperactivity (Grades 0 to 4), palpable pulmonary second or mitral first sound (Grades 0 to 4).

(5) *Auscultation diagram* (Figure 1.1) of sound events in apex and aortic or pulmonary area, grades, increased sounds, and clicks and snaps 0–4 for intensity, marking thrill with 'T' and murmurs 0–4 for intensity above the diagram and 0–4 for duration below it.

Investigations

(1) *ECG*: summarize main features – rate, rhythm, axis, P wave, P–R interval, Q wave, QRS complex with bundle blocks, S–T segment and T wave with comment on exercise effect if done, and the heights of R and S waves in leads V_1 and V_5 (Figures 1.2 and 1.3).

(2) *Chest X-rays*: a p–a, penetrated p–a, and penetrated lateral with

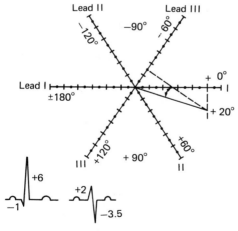

Figure 1.2 Measurement of axis deviation. The algebraical sum of the positive and negative deflections of QRS in standard lead is plotted in arbitrary units, along the axis of lead III. Perpendiculars are dropped and a line drawn from the centre of the triaxial system to their point of intersection

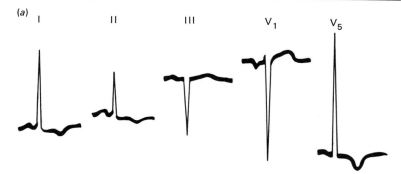

Tall R waves over left ventricle. R > 25 mm in V_5; S > 25 mm in V_1; R V × SV_5 < 35 mm. Strain pattern of S–T in left ventricular leads.

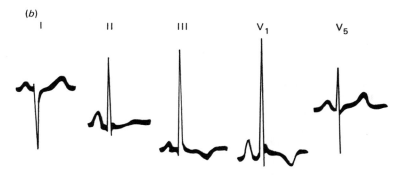

Tall R waves and strain pattern in right ventricular leads. R > S in V_1 or R > 8 mm in V_1.

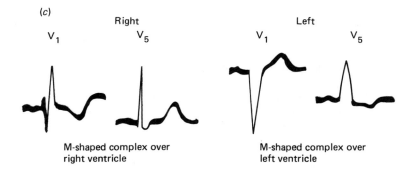

M-shaped complex over right ventricle

M-shaped complex over left ventricle

Figure 1.3 (*a*) Left ventricular hypertrophy; (*b*) right ventricular hypertrophy; (*c*) bundle branch block – QRS wider than 0.12 s

film on left should be examined for cardiothoracic ratio, chamber enlargement (0–4), of ascending aorta, right atrium, inferior cava, subclavian, aortic knuckle, pulmonary artery, main pulmonary vessels, left atrial appendage, ventricular mass. On the penetrated p–a the left atrium and on the lateral the presence of calcification of mitral or aortic valves, coronary arteries or ductus, and the identification of which ventricle is enlarged. Pulmonary disease and Kerley's lines in the lung fields and the presence of abnormalities of the chest wall should also be identified.

(3) *Catheter and angiographic data*: oxygen step-ups, gradients, pulmonary hypertension, exercise or other provocative tests giving positive results, angiographic demonstration of stenoses, shunts, myopathies, anatomical abnormalities and coronary artery disease.

(4) *Blood*: haemoglobin, ESR, full blood count, platelets, coagulation screen, grouping, cross matching, liver function, cardiac enzymes, urea, electrolytes, creatinine clearance, magnesium, T3 test if in atrial fibrillation, lipids, cholesterol, HB_sAg and HIV screen.

(5) Cultures of urine, throat swab, nasal swab, sputum, perineal skin.

(6) Respiratory function tests.

(7) Dental inspection including X-rays for unsuspected roots or periapical or periodontal disease.

(8) Psychiatric interview if indicated.

(9) Height and weight must be recorded and daily weighing commenced.

Pre-operative treatment

(1) Treat any block or multiple bundle branch block by pacing, total body potassium deficit with extra potassium and spironolactone; digitalization and diuretic-induced dehydration by stopping drugs in time. Beta blockade by stopping drugs at a suitable time (not at all in angina).

(2) All patients should be regarded as germ carriers and given antiseptic baths and antiseptic shampoos, from which they go to completely freshly laundered linen, eschew linen handkerchiefs, use nasal antiseptic cream, and avoid postoperative patients.

(3) Relatives must be seen before surgery and the risk–cost benefit analysis described and the operation and postoperative course explained, with a visit to the intensive care ward if possible. The

patient should be made familiar with the intensive care ward and its routine as far as possible.

(4) Physiotherapy: the routine of exercise for lungs and limbs should be thoroughly imbued in the patient before operation, and the rationale of ventilation, the possibility of its use and a trial of how it feels should be given.

(5) Antibiotics: various regimes exist. There seems no argument about the necessity for prophylactic antibiotics in open heart patients for at least the three peri-operative days (until all tubes and drips are removed) and possibly for two weeks (in patients with prosthetic valves). Subsequent antibiotics should be specific therapeutic weapons dictated by laboratory cultures.

(6) Other treatment: maintenance therapy of patients with Addison disease, steroid treatment, diabetes, hypothyroidism, gout and epilepsy, pancreatic deficiency, other forms of malabsorption, allergies, arthritis, vitamin deficiencies and pernicious anaemia, should have careful maintenance over the surgical period by consultation with the physician treating the condition normally.

(7) Beta blockers: these lower oxygen demand but do so by lowering myocardial contractility which could prejudice postoperative recovery. This danger has been exaggerated in the past and we know now that beta blockers improve peroperative myocardial preservation with little diminution of myocardial work capacity, only some alteration in the violence with which that work is done. The net effect may be to have a more contractile heart in the postoperative phase if beta blockade was adequate before peroperative global ischaemia. Moreover, the beta adrenergic tachycardia may reduce ventricular efficiency, especially in the presence of pathological ventricles or mechanical prosthetic valves, so that beta blockade may increase cardiac efficiency.

(8) Calcium antagonists: these generally inhibit conduction rather than contraction within the myocardium and relax the plain muscle of the coronary vasculature. They are also known, however, to protect the myocardium against global ischaemia such as is used during heart operations and thus the patient may return to the ITU better from having had adequate protection of this sort. The administration of verapamil to someone who is fully beta blocked may however produce fatal asystole.

(9) Aspirin: many patients may need aspirin for its antiplatelet effect in subtotal coronary occlusion. This effect takes about

two weeks to wear off and surgery in some cases should be delayed until this interval has elapsed if possible.

(10) Isosorbide dinitrate, other nitrates and other peripheral vaso-dilators such as the alpha blockers have all been wrongly feared in the past when the patient's pressure was thought to reflect his well-being. By reducing the peripheral resistance and hence the afterload against which the compromised ventricle is working, they increase cardiac output and tissue perfusion and at the same time reduce the venous pressure on both sides of the heart, so improving the transcapillary pressure gradient and lowering the mean capillary pressure and thus the tissue oedema with its attendant resistance to the passage of gases and nutrients. The heart benefits particularly from these improved substrate dynamics. A factor which militated against the use of nitrites intravenously in the past was their instability in solution. This technical problem has now been overcome. A starting dose of 1 mg over 10 min in an intravenous solution is used, and it is important to maintain reasonable filling press-ures when the effect appears, as too low a filling pressure is as bad for ventricular output as too high a filling pressure is for capillary effectiveness.

Emergency situations

It may be necessary to undertake treatment of patients dying of acute cardiogenic shock from pulmonary emboli or myocardial infarction. In either case investigations must be done to make precise surgical treatment possible. The pulmonary angiogram for emboli may prove fatal without supportive veno–arterial pump oxygenator bypass, and the coronary angiography for myocardial pre-infarction patients similarly may necessitate balloon counterpulsation.

The indications for these supportive techniques and the procedure and management of them should be well known by all staff concerned with these emergencies. Essentially, their use is indicated when low output shock continues to worsen despite full inotropic support and correction of metabolic acidosis, blood gas and electro-lyte abnormalities.

Emergency admissions

(1) *Previously known patients*. These patients should be admitted under their previous consultant if the reason for admission is the condition that consultant was treating, and subject to the firm in question being available and agreeable. If this is not the case, the

admission should be to the firm 'on take', and the patient passed back to his previous consultant the next day.

(2) *New cases.*

(a) Non-traumatic. These patients will be admitted to the duty firm, and the consultant fully appraised of the situation when all the necessary clarification has been done.

(b) Traumatic. In the absence of proof to the contrary, all organs and body cavities must be suspected of having suffered injury, especially in high velocity motor vehicle accidents. Even a slow and seemingly gentle thoracic crush injury may be associated with serious abdominal or pelvic damage. Consultation with abdominal and neurosurgeons should be early in these patients.

Shock

Shock is a clinical syndrome of tissue hypoperfusion, cellular hypoxia and acute metabolic impairment with damage to vital organs.

There are four main types of shock:

(1) Cardiogenic (pump);
(2) Hypovolaemic (fluid);
(3) Vasogenic (peripheral resistance);
(4) Septic (mixed).

Cardiogenic shock may be caused by ischaemic heart disease, arrhythmias, open heart surgery, cardiac tamponade, myocardial disease or heart valve malfunction.

Hypovolaemic shock could be caused by haemorrhage, fluid sequestration (pancreatitis, burns), or extracellular fluid loss (vomiting, diarrhoea, enteric fistulae).

Vasogenic shock may result from spinal anaesthesia, anaphylaxis, excess of vasodilators.

Septic shock is a complicated condition with a combination of fluid maldistribution, poor tissue metabolism, cardiac depression and vasomotor instability.

The hypoperfusion and cellular anoxia (common findings to any form of shock) damage the cell progressively and lead to death or multisystem failure. Early signs are low systolic pressure, respiratory alkalosis and dry skin. Later, lower blood pressure, oliguria, metabolic acidosis and peripheral hypoperfusion with neurological signs may be present.

Every type of shock must be treated on its merits. Nevertheless, a general therapeutic target might be:

- Cardiac index at 4.0–5.5 l/min/m²
- MAP over 80 mmHg or systolic over 100 mmHg
- PAWP below 25 mmHg
- Pao_2 above 60 mmHg or 8 kPa
- pH between 7.34 and 7.48
- Oxygen consumption above 170–200 ml/min/m²
- Haematocrit between 25 and 35%
- Blood volume above 500 ml in excess of predictive values
- Diuresis 0.5–1.0 ml/kg/h
- CVP lower than 15 cmH₂O
- Sinus rhythm

Cardiorespiratory arrest

This is the lack of an effective pulse and tissue perfusion and/or lack of ventilation of the lung with poor blood oxygenation predisposed to by acidosis, cardiac, respiratory, renal or hepatic insufficiency, hypersedation, cerebrovascular accidents, surgery or trauma to the thoracic cage, cardiac arrhythmias, toxic or septic insult. The brain has 95% aerobic metabolism, requiring 775 ml/min at basal level, which at rest is 15–20% of cardiac output. Very short ischaemic periods are followed by oedema of the brain with further inhibition of perfusion.

The ABC of resuscitation is:

A . . . Airways
B . . . Breathing
C . . . Circulation
D . . . Drugs
E . . . ECG monitoring
F . . . Fibrillation control

And all these should be achieved simultaneously.

Airways: should be cleared (Figures 1.4–1.6) – remember the Heimlich manoeuvre for bolus occlusion of the pharynx. The tongue should be kept from falling into the airway (Figure 1.7).
Breathing: ventilation mouth to mouth, by mask, by cannula, by endotracheal tube (Figure 1.8), mini-tracheostomy or tracheostomy.
Circulation: precordial blow may produce a pulse in a temporarily asystolic heart. If not, massage at 70–80 beats/min, concomitant

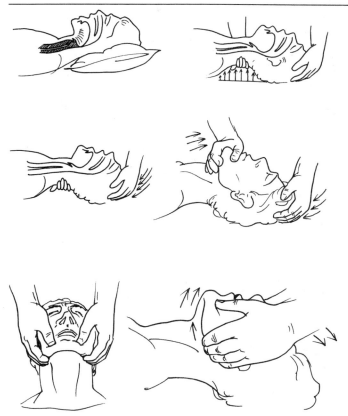

Figure 1.4 Basic manoeuvres to avoid airway obstruction

with ventilation, will produce ejection in either asystole or ventricular fibrillation (Figure 1.9).

Drugs: an intravenous route is essential. Depending on anoxic time, the appropriate medication is given.

- Adrenaline: 0.5–2.0 mg every 5 min if necessary.
  Infusion: 0.02–0.2 µg/kg/min
- Noradrenaline: 0.5–1.0 mg every 5 min if necessary.
  Infusion: 0.01–0.2 µg/kg/min
- Dopamine: Infusion 2–20 µg/kg/min
- Dobutamine: Infusion 2–20 µg/kg/min
- Calcium chloride: 2.0–5.0 mmol

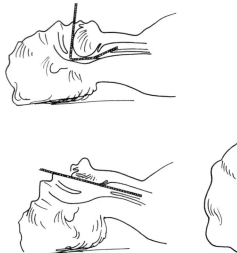

Figure 1.5 Lifting neck up will correct the angle mouth–airways

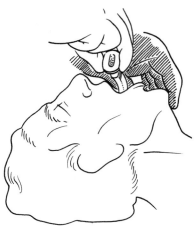

Figure 1.6 An airway is inserted into the mouth

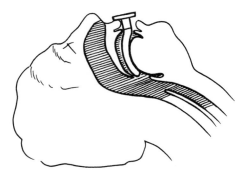

Figure 1.7 Position of the airway preventing the tongue from occluding the larynx

- Atropine: 0.2–2.0 mg
- Bicarbonate: 1 mmol/kg initial dose. Then 0.5 mmol/kg every 5 min of arrest until gases indicate different doses.
- Lignocaine: 1 mg/kg initial dose.
                Infusion: 2–4 mg/min

ECG monitoring is vital to distinguish asystole, ventricular fibrilla-

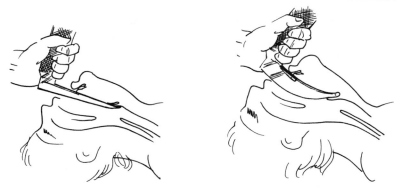

Figure 1.8 Two different types of endotracheal intubation with straight and curved laryngoscopes

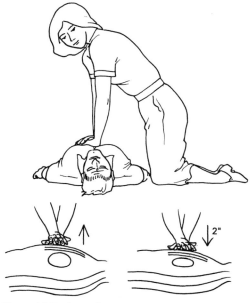

Figure 1.9 Basic cardiac massage

tion, electromechanical dissociation or particular arrhythmias to be treated.

Ventricular fibrillation should be shocked first, then treated specifically. If no monitor is available, defibrillation should be performed first.

ATRIAL FIBRILLATION
Artrial rate 350—600/min
Ventricular rate 120/min
irregularly irregular

ATRIAL FLUTTER
Atrial rate 200—400/min
Ventricles 110/min
2 : 1 block.

ATRIAL TACHYCARDIA
Last 3 complexes SR.
Ventricles regular 120/min
during paroxysm.

VENTRICULAR
TACHYCARDIA
P waves unrelated to ventricles
Bizarre ventricular complexes.

1st DEGREE HEART
BLOCK
P—R interval > 0.21 s

2nd DEGREE HEART
BLOCK
Wenckebach gives increasing
P—R interval till beat dropped.
May show only dropped beats.

3rd DEGREE HEART
BLOCK
Complete A—V dissociation.
Atrial rate 70—80/min
Ventricular rate 20—40/min

WOLFF-PARKINSON-
WHITE
P—R interval short. QRS wide
due to delta waves.

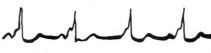

Figure 1.10 Arrhythmias

Cardiac arrhythmias (Figure 1.10)

There are two main mechanisms for arrhythmias:

(1) Enhanced automaticity;
(2) Re-entry.

Some characteristics of common arrhythmias are shown in Table 1.1.

Table 1.1

Type	Ventricular rate (beats/min)	A:V ratio	Special features
Sinus arrhythmia	100–150	1:1	Normal P wave. Irregular rate (varying with respiration)
Paroxysmal supraventricular tachycardia (SVT)	150–200	1:1	Look for WPW (delta waves)
Ectopic atrial tachycardia	100–150	1:1–3:1	Abnormal P wave
Atrial flutter	140–160	2:1–4:1	Saw-tooth pattern
Atrial fibrillation	120–180	–	Irregular R–R
1st degree block	Variable	1:1	PR interval > 200 ms
2nd degree block			
Type I	Variable	2:3–4:5	Gradual PR increase (Wenckebach)
Type II	Variable	2:1–4:1	PR interval fixed
3rd degree block	–	–	No A–V conduct
Junctional tachycardia	80–140	–	Absent P wave
Ventricular tachycardia	100–200	–	Leads to VF
Ventricular fibrillation	–	–	Cardiac arrest

Anti-arrhythmic drugs

Class I. Membrane stabilizing; reduce conductivity, excitability and automaticity

Subgroup IA – moderate reduction in conductivity and prolongation of action potential duration.

(1) Quinidine
* Indications: ventricular arrhythmias.
* Dose by mouth: 200–400 mg 3–4 times daily.
* Side effects: diarrhoea, thrombocytopenia, haemolytic anaemia. Also, prolongs the QT interval and may lead to torsade de pointes.

* Contraindications: heart block.
(2) Procainamide
   * Indications: ventricular arrhythmias.
   * Dose: by mouth: 250 mg 4–6 times daily.
            i.v. injection: 25–50 mg/min, max. 1 g.
   * Side effects: diarrhoea, fever, lupus erythematosus-like syndrome, QT interval prolongation.
   * Contraindications: heart block, heart failure.

(3) Disopyramide
   * Indications: post-MI ventricular arrhythmias.
   * Dose: by mouth: 300–800 mg daily
            i.v. injection: 2 mg/kg over 5 min followed by oral dose of 200 mg.
            i.v. infusion: 400 μg/kg/h to max. 800 mg daily.
   * Side effects: hypotension, severe anticholinergic effects, QT interval prolongation.
   * Contraindications: heart block, heart failure, glaucoma.

Subgroup IB – depression of automaticity, reduction of amplitudes or delayed after-depolarization with increased VF threshold.

(1) Lignocaine
   * Indications: ventricular ectopics – more than 8 per minute, multifocal, runs of VT, ectopic on T wave, haemodynamic impairment.
   * Dose: 1 mg/kg initial dose, followed by infusion of 1–4 mg/min.
   * Side effects: CNS signs (convulsions).
   * Contraindications: liver failure, severe low cardiac output, heart block.

(2) Mexiletine
   * Indications: ventricular arrhythmias.
   * Dose: by mouth: 400 mg initially, followed by 200 mg after 2 h and 3–4 times daily.
            i.v. injection: 25 mg/min for 5–10 min, followed by infusion of 250 mg/h for 1 h and 125 mg for 2 h.
   * Contraindications: heart block.

(3) Tocainide
   * Indications: severe and refractory ventricular arrythmias.
   * Dose: by mouth: 400 mg 3 times a day.
            i.v. injection: 500 mg over 30 min followed by oral dose.

* Side effects: CNS signs, nausea, aplastic anaemia, fibrosing alveolitis.
* Contraindications: severe renal or hepatic failure, heart block.

(4) Phenytoin
   * Indications: digitalis-induced arrhythmias.
   * Dose: by mouth: 300–400 mg/day.
      i.v. injection: 3–5 mg/kg over 10 min.
   * Side effects: CNS symptoms, hypotension.
   * Contraindications: SVT, heart block.

Subgroup IC – do not prolong ventricular repolarization period; prolong QRS.

(1) Flecainide
   * Indications: ventricular arrhythmias.
   * Dose: by mouth: 100–200 mg 12-hourly
      i.v. injection: 2 mg/kg over 30 min.
      i.v. infusion: 250 µg/kg/h
   * Side effects: nausea, dizziness.
   * Contraindications: heart failure, heart block.

(2) Encainide

(3) Lorcainide

Class II. Beta blockers

(1) Beta-1 selective: Acebutolol
                      Atenolol
                      Metoprolol

(2) Non-selective: Propranolol
                   Oxprenolol
                   Sotalol
                   Nadolol
                   Timolol
                   Pindolol

(3) Beta and alpha effects: Labetalol

Class III. Repolarization prolongers

(1) Amiodarone
   * Indications: WPW syndrome, refractory supraventricular arrhythmias.

* Dose: by mouth: 200 mg 8-hourly for one week, followed by 200 mg 12-hourly for one week and then 200 mg daily.
  i.v. injection: 5 mg/kg over 1–2 h
* Side effects: neuropathy, thyroid dysfunction, hepatitis, CNS signs, corneal microdeposits.
* Contraindications: heart block, pregnancy.

(2) Bretylium
* Indications: refractory ventricular arrhythmia.
* Dose: i.m. injection: 5 mg/kg 1 dose
  i.v. injection: 5–10 mg/kg over 10 min.
  Infusion: 1–2 mg/min.
* Side effects: nausea, hypotension.

Class IV. Calcium antagonists

(1) Verapamil
* Indications: supraventricular tachyarrhythmias.
* Dose: by mouth: 40–120 mg 8-hourly.
  i.v. injection: 5–10 mg over 5–10 min.
* Side effects: vomiting, bradycardia, hypotension.
* Contraindications: heart block, heart failure.

(2) Nifedipine

(3) Diltiazem

Pacemakers

Definitions

Pulse generator: Source of energy and circuits.
Lead: Wire from the pulse generator to the electrode.
Electrode: Tip of the lead in contact with myocardium (epicardium or endocardium).
Unipolar pacing: Negative electrode in the myocardium and positive electrode distant from the heart.
Negative electrode: Stimulating pole of the system.
Positive electrode: Ground pole of the system.
Bipolar pacing: Negative and positive electrodes in the myocardium.
Endocardial pacing: i.v. pacing. Electrode in the endocardium.
Epicardial pacing: Surgical pacing. Electrode in the epicardium.
Stimulating threshold: Minimal amount of current that will stimulate the myocardium.

Resistance: Combined resistance electrode-myocardium-lead.

Measures: Volt = Voltage threshold
milliAmps = Current threshold
Ohms = Resistance

Types of pacemaker generators

(1) *Asynchronous*: The circuit just forms electrical impulses. Competes with the patient's own electrical activity and may cause VT. Consumes energy.
(2) *Synchronous*: Two circuits – one forms impulses, one acts as a sensing circuit. The system may be inhibited or stimulated by the wave.
(3) *Sequential*: Preserves A–V contraction sequence.
(4) *Programmable*: Mainly rate, output, R wave sensitivity, refractory periods, PR interval, synchronicity.

Nomenclature

Three letter code:

First = Chamber paced (A,V,D)
Second = Chamber sensed (A,V,D,O)
Third = Mode of generator action
(Inhibited, Triggered, Asynchronous)

Thus:
VOO = Pacing the ventricle. Asynchronous.
AOO = Pacing the atrium.
VVI = Pacing and sensing the ventricle. Inhibited by ventricular electrical activity.
DVI = Atrium and ventricle paced. Inhibited by R waves.
DDD = Completely automatic.

Indications for permanent pacing

- Sick sinus syndrome.
- Symptomatic second degree Möbitz type II heart block.
- Symptomatic sinus bradycardia refractory to treatment.
- Acquired complete heart block.
- Recurrent ventricular fibrillation (implantable defibrillator).

Indications for temporary pacing

- Drug-associated symptomatic bradycardia.
- Second degree Möbitz type II heart block after MI.

- Symptomatic bifascicular block.
- Postoperative period of heart surgery if heart block has been present during the operation.
- Mitral valve replacement.

Heart failure

Heart failure is the result of the inability of the heart to pump enough blood to the tissues for normal metabolic functions.
It can be caused by:

(1) *Increased afterload*: aortic stenosis, hypertension, pulmonary stenosis, pulmonary hypertension.
(2) *Increased preload*: aortic incompetence, mitral incompetence, ASD, VSD, pulmonary valve incompetence, tricuspid valve incompetence.
(3) *Myocardial damage*: ischaemic heart disease, myocarditis, congestive cardiomyopathy.
(4) *Excessively high output*: systemic shunts, hyperthyroidism, pulmonary emphysema.

The heart compensates by increasing the rate, ventricular dilatation, ventricular hypertrophy and arterial vasoconstriction.

Left heart failure with increased left atrial pressure will cause dyspnoea, orthopnoea, nocturnal dyspnoea or pulmonary oedema from pulmonary venous congestion and exercise-induced cough, bronchitis and haemoptysis from bronchial venous congestion. The right heart may fail from left heart-induced pulmonary hypertension as well as disorders of the right heart.

Once a thorough physical examination, ECG and chest X-rays and laboratory tests have been performed, echocardiogram will show valve function, ejection fraction and myocardial contractility. Angiography will rule out three main causes: valve, coronary or myocardial disease.

Treatment is the alleviation of the causative mechanism. The failing myocardium can be helped by reducing its afterload and stabilizing its rhythm and rate to the most efficient.

Systemic demand can be minimized by rest and weight reduction; if excessive, pulmonary congestion may then be palliated with sodium restriction and diuretics. Inotropics may usefully improve myocardial contractility.

Functional status may be classified as follows:

Class I: Normal activity. Prevented by symptoms from athletic activity.

Class II: A – Prevented from hurrying.
            B – Prevented from normal walking.
Class III: Prevented from even slow walking.
Class IV: Complete limitation. Symptomatic at rest.

Inotropics used in heart failure

(1) *Cardiac glycosides* (heart failure with fast rate from atrial fibrillation) – see Table 1.2.

Table 1.2

Drug	Onset (min)	Peak effect (h)	Dose
Digoxin	15–30	2–5	Urgent: 1.0–1.5 mg in 24 h Elective: 0.25 mg/day for 3–6 days Maintenance: 0.25–0.5 mg/day
Digitoxin	25–120	4–12	50–200 µg/day
Ouabain	5–10	0.5–2	Up to 1 mg i.v. slowly

(2) *Beta-1 adrenoreceptor drugs* (see Section on Inotropics used in intensive care, p. 58).

- Adrenaline
- Noradrenaline
- Isoprenaline
- Dopamine
- Dobutamine
- Prenalterol

(3) *Beta-2 adrenoreceptor drugs*

- Salbutamol
- Terbutaline
- Pirbuterol

Vasodilators used in heart failure

(A) Direct acting
(1) Nitrates, e.g. glyceryl trinitrate.
   * Dose: Sublingual: 0.5–1.0 mg prn.
            Oral: 2–6 mg 8–12-hourly.
            i.v.: 10–200 µg/min.

(2) Hydralazine
* Dose: Oral: 25–50 mg 12-hourly
i.v.: 20–40 mg slowly

(B) Neurohumoral
(1) Prazosin
* Dose: Oral: 500 µg initially and 1 mg 6–8-hourly.
Maintenance: 4–10 mg/day

(2) Captopril
* Dose: Oral: 25–50 mg 8–12-hourly.

(3) Others
 ● Regitine
 ● Dibenyline
 ● Priscol
 ● Diazoxide

(C) Calcium channel antagonists
(1) Nifedipine
* Dose: 5–20 mg 8-hourly.

(2) Verapamil
* 80–240 mg 12-hourly.

(3) Diltiazem
* Dose: 60 mg 8-hourly.

Acute pulmonary oedema

Pulmonary overload secondary to heart failure is balanced initially
by increased lymph drainage. Afterwards, fluid accumulates into the
lung interstitium and then into the alveolar spaces, causing respiratory distress, deterioration of blood gases and chest X-ray signs.
Other causes of pulmonary oedema are usually related to damage to
the alveolo-capillary membrane, with intra-alveolar oedema.
   The cause must first be determined and the following initial
treatment given.

(1) Morphine (i.m. or i.v.) 2–10 mg, except in cases of chronic
obstructive airway disease. It increases vasodilatation of pulmonary vasculature and calms the patient.
(2) 100% oxygen under positive pressure.
(3) Sitting position and rotating tourniquets.

(4) Intravenous diuretics, e.g. frusemide, 40–120 mg. It reduces circulating volume and dilates the venous system.
(5) Vasodilators, e.g. glyceryl trinitrate, 0.4 mg every 3–5 min. In extreme cases, sodium nitroprusside at 5–20 µg/kg/min.
(6) Digoxin, 0.5–0.75 mg i.v. initial dose or ouabain up to 1 mg, or lanatoside C, 1.5 mg i.v.
(7) Aminophylline, 240–480 mg i.v. reduces bronchoconstriction, increases sodium excretion and diuresis. Also, increases cardiac contractility.
(8) Mechanical ventilation if pH less than 7.1, $P\text{CO}_2$ higher than 70 mmHg (9.3 kPa), $P\text{O}_2$ lower than 60 mmHg (8 kPa) if high oxygen concentration is already given.
(9) Intra-aortic balloon pump helps in cases of non-hypertensive pulmonary oedema refractory to medical treatment.

Hypertensive emergencies

Some of the hypertensive emergencies encountered are:
(a) hypertensive encephalopathy;
(b) acute aortic dissection;
(c) central nervous system bleeding;
(d) acute left ventricular failure;
(e) myocardial infarction with persistent pain and sustained hypertension;
(f) accelerated malignant hypertension;
(g) eclampsia;
(h) acute renal failure;
(i) retinal haemorrhage;
(j) postoperative bleeding especially after or during emergency surgery, open heart surgery, renal transplantation and phaeochromocytoma.

The treatment conventionally aims to lower the diastolic blood pressure down to levels around 90 mmHg. The main drugs used are shown in Table 1.3.

Table 1.3

Drug	Dose	Onset	Duration
Diazoxide	150–300 mg	1–3 min	4–12 h
Nitroprusside	1–20 µg/kg/min	1 min	2–5 min
Trimetaphan	1–15 mg/min	1 min	2–5 min
Hydralazine	10–20 mg every 10 min	10–20 min	2–6 h
Methyldopa	500 mg over 30 min	1–3 h	2–12 h
Reserpine		2–3 h	6–24 h

Other drugs are:

- Isosorbide (2–10 mg/h)
- Glyceryl trinitrate (10–200 μg/min)
- Labetalol (1 mg/kg/h)
- Propranolol (1 mg every 2 min up to 10 mg)
- Phentolamine (0.1–2.0 mg/min up to 60 mg)
- Phenoxybenzamine (1–2 mg/kg daily in two divided doses)
- Captopril (12.5 mg 12-hourly)
- Enalapril (2.5–20 mg/day)
- Largactil (25–50 mg 6–8-hourly)

Special contraindications to these drugs are:

- Myocardial infarction
- Cerebral ischaemia
- Heart block

Coronary circulation

From the surgical viewpoint, there are four major trunk or branch coronary arteries (Figure 1.11):

(a) left main;
(b) left anterior descendant (LAD);
(c) left circumflex;
(d) right coronary artery.

The atrioventricular circle is formed by the right and the circumflex, and the interventricular circle by the LAD and the posterior descending branch of the right coronary. The back of the heart is supplied by obtuse marginals from the circumflex and the front of the heart by diagonals and septal branches from the LAD system. Laterally, both the LAD and the circumflex irrigate the myocardium.

The artery which supplies the posterior descending (the PDA) is called 'dominant'. For instance, if the PDA comes from the right coronary, then the heart has dominant right. If the PDA comes from the circumflex, the heart has dominant left.

Surgically, the left main stem can be located between the pulmonary artery and the left atrial appendage. After 5–10 mm it divides into LAD (anterior interventricular groove) and circumflex (posterior atrioventricular groove and posterior interventricular groove for

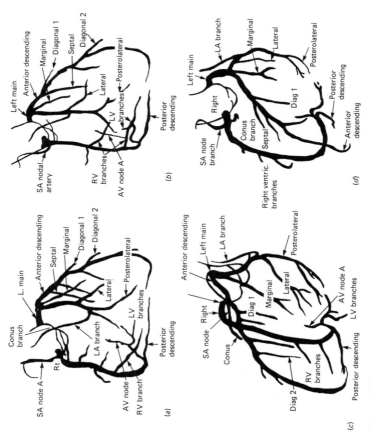

Figure 1.11 Anatomic representation of the coronary arteries: (*a*) anteroposterior; (*b*) right anterior oblique; (*c*) lateral; (*d*) left anterior oblique

its branches). The right coronary artery runs in the atrioventricular groove and then laterally to the right, giving off a sino-atrial nodal, atrioventricular nodal, right ventricular branches and the posterior descending artery.

The venous system goes to the coronary sinus in the postero-inferior atrioventricular groove, formed by the great cardiac vein (accompanying the anterior descending artery), the oblique vein (from the left atrium) and the middle cardiac vein (accompanying the posterior descending artery).

Ischaemic heart disease

An inadequate myocardial perfusion from coronary obstruction leads to impaired tissue oxygenation and, if acute, to tissue necrosis (myocardial infarction).

Increased risk factors in angina pectoris are:
- left ventricular dysfunction;
- previous ischaemic episodes;
- cardiomegaly;
- poor treadmill performance.

Severe ischaemia is signified by:
- dyspnoea;
- unstable angina;
- resting ECG changes;
- severe ECG changes during the acute attack;
- early symptoms on treadmill;
- poor response to medical therapy.

Predisposing risk factors are:
- age;
- hypertension;
- inactivity;
- smoking;
- lipid alterations associated with obesity.

Angiographically, adverse factors are:
- left ventricular dysfunction;
- left main stem obstruction;
- multiple vessel disease;
- proximal occlusion of an important vessel;
- poor distal vessels.

Anginal pain is retrosternal, oppressive, radiating to neck, arms and epigastrium, worse with meals, emotion, exertion and cold weather. It should also be remembered that other diseases may produce angina even in the presence of normal coronary arteries (aortic stenosis, mitral stenosis, severe hypertension, anaemia, hyperthyroidism and bradyarrhythmias).

The initial treatment of angina is based on control of precipitating factors, becoming thin and normotensive and stopping smoking completely. Then, drug treatment is started.

(1) *Beta blockers* (reduce myocardial oxygen demand)
- Atenolol (Tenormin): 25–200 mg
- Propranolol (Inderal): 80–360 mg
- Nadolol (Corgard): 20–320 mg
- Metoprolol (Lopresor): 50–200 mg
- Pindolol (Visken): 7.5–22.5 mg
- Timolol (Blocadren): 10–40 mg
- Acebutolol (Sectral): 400–1200 mg
- Labetalol (Trandate): 300–1200 mg
* Contraindications: severe left ventricular dysfunction, asthma, sinus bradycardia, severe chronic obstructive airways disease.

(2) *Calcium channel blockers* (reduce afterload and improve coronary spasm)
- Diltiazem (Tildiem): 120–360 mg
- Nifedipine (Adalat): 30–120 mg
- Verapamil (Cordilox): 240–480 mg

(3) *Nitrates* (reduce preload, afterload and coronary tone)
- Glyceryl trinitrate: 5.2–19.2 mg/day (sublingual: 0.3–1.0 mg prn)
- Isosorbide dinitrate: 30–120 mg/day (sublingual: 5–10 mg prn)
- Isosorbide mononitrate: 20–120 mg/day
- Pentaerythritol tetranitrate: 60–240 mg/day

Indications for coronary angiography

The main indications for coronary angiography are:

(a) unstable angina;
(b) incapacitating angina;
(c) suspected left main obstruction;
(d) valve disease and angina;
(e) unexplained heart failure;
(f) post-infarction angina;

(g) post-infarction complications (septal rupture, mitral incompe-
    tence, ventricular aneurysm, sustained and refractory VT);
(h) severe low cardiac output post-infarction;
(i) congenital anomalies in the coronaries;
(j) persistent angina with non-conclusive tests;
(k) post-thrombolytic therapy for MI.

From the point of view of the exercise test, indications for
angiography are:

(a) early, severe, persistent, extensive ST changes;
(b) a fall in the blood pressure.

The most important surgical indications in ischaemic heart disease are:

(a) coronary obstruction with symptoms despite full medical ther-
    apy;
(b) left main stem obstruction;
(c) post-infarction obstruction with angina;
(d) coronary occlusion and sustained ventricular tachycardia;
(e) post-infarction complications;
(f) coronary disease associated with other surgical heart disease
    such as aortic stenosis.

Emergency treatment

Unstable angina is deteriorating ischaemic heart disease with
increased risk of myocardial infarction and death, characterized by
angina at rest, lasting longer than 20 min and unresponsive to
enteral therapy.

Once myocardial infarction is ruled out and the patient sedated
and on full treatment (i.v. nitroglycerin, beta blockers, calcium
channel blockers, antiplatelets), if the patient remains unstable,
insertion of an intra-aortic balloon before angiography may be
advisable. Otherwise angiography is performed as an emergency. If
there is single vessel disease without calcification, percutaneous
transluminal coronary angioplasty (PTCA) is attempted. If there are
more vessels involved, if there is intravascular calcification, or if
obstructions are eccentric or at important branchings, surgery is the
best option.

PTCA has been performed since 1977. It is advisable to have a
coronary surgery team available. This technique can be used in
single vessel disease with angina pectoris, after thrombolytic therapy
for myocardial infarction and in acute unstable angina. Complica-

tions include coronary occlusion, dissection, thrombosis, arrhythmias and re-stenosis after dilatation.

Myocardial infarction

In myocardial infarction the prognosis is related to the extent of the necrosis, associated clinical conditions and complications of the acute episode. There may be tachycardia, arrhythmias, hypotension and low cardiac output.

The ECG shows ST elevation in the acute phase, Q waves and T inversion afterwards (Figure 1.12). If the necrosis is present in the inferior surface (right coronary artery), ECG signs will be found in leads II, III and aVF; if the infarction compromises the anteroseptal area, signs will be present in V_1–V_4 (left anterior descending artery); when the lateral wall is involved, the abnormalities will be detected in leads I, aVL, V_5 and V_6 (circumflex artery).

Management of myocardial infarction

The initial management of non-complicated myocardial infarction is to relieve pain, maintain an adequate intravenous line, control arrhythmias, and treat cardiac arrest or low cardiac output. If the patient is stable, the first medications given may be:

- Morphine (5–15 mg i.v.) unless advanced respiratory disease is present;
- Glyceryl trinitrate infusion (25–200 µg/kg/min);
- Diazepam (5–10 mg i.m., oral)

Ventricular arrhythmias can be controlled with lignocaine, 1 mg/kg i.v. bolus followed by infusion at 1–4 mg/min if necessary.

Early treatment of *heart failure* is with inotropics (see section on Inotropics in intensive care, p. 58). *Anticoagulation* is necessary if there are suspicions of thrombus in the left ventricle or deep venous thrombosis or embolism are present. Prophylactic heparin is given subcutaneously at 5000 units 8–12-hourly.

Most patients receive beta blockers unless heart failure or bradycardia complicate the situation (usually metoprolol, 100 mg twice a day), and if hypertension is associated with the infarction, sodium nitroprusside infusion is commenced at 1–15 µg/kg/min.

If the patient is seen within 4 h of the acute attack, intravenous streptokinase (1 million units over 30 min) will reduce the infarct size. If the pain subsides, medical treatment is continued. Otherwise the patient is taken for cineangiography and the choice between

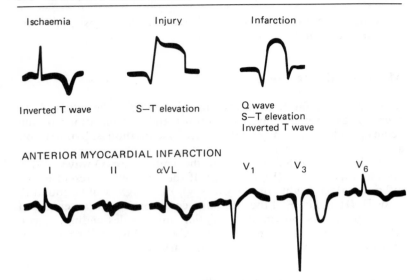

ANTERIOR MYOCARDIAL INFARCTION

Typical infarct pattern in leads I, αVL and precordial leads.

INFERIOR MYOCARDIAL INFARCTION

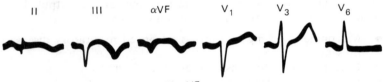

Typical infarct pattern in leads II, III, αVF.

TRUE POSTERIOR MYOCARDIAL INFARCTION

True posterior infarction results in tall R waves in leads V_1 and V_2 and diagnosis is one of exclusion of other causes. These are : right ventricular hypertrophy, right bundle branch block, and the Wolff-Parkinson-White syndrome.

AGE OF THE INFARCT

During the weeks following acute infarction the S—T elevation gradually returns to the baseline and at that time tall, symmetrical T waves appear in leads facing the uninjured surface. Following this the T waves gradually return to normal and the only remaining evidence of previous infarction is an abnormal Q wave.

Should the pattern of acute infarction remain longer than 6 months it is suggestive of ventricular aneurysm.

Figure 1.12 Myocardial infarction in lead placed over damaged muscle

intracoronary streptokinase, percutaneous transluminal coronary angioplasty or coronary surgery is made according to each unit's experience and results.

A Swan-Ganz catheter may be inserted and pulmonary capillary wedge pressure (PCWP) should be maintained between 14 and 18 mmHg and left ventricular end diastolic pressure (LVEDP) between 20 and 24 mmHg. With these numbers, some clinical diagnoses may be supported as follows:

- Low CVP and low PCWP suggest hypovolaemia.
- PCWP > CVP;   CVP/PCWP < 0.65;   PAEDP = PCWP suggests left ventricular failure.
- CVP > PCWP; CVP/PCWP > 0.65; PAEDP > PCWP supports diagnosis of pulmonary embolism.
- CVP = PCWP; PAEDP = PCWP strongly suggests cardiac tamponade.

Complicated myocardial infarction

Cardiogenic shock may be defined numerically as:

- Systolic pressure lower than 80 mmHg (10.7 kPa)
- PCWP higher than 18 mmHg (2.4 kPa)
- Cardiac index lower than 2 l/min/m^2 (associated with clinical signs of low cardiac output).

It must be remembered that a low blood pressure results from arrhythmias, hypovolaemia, right ventricular infarct, left ventricular failure, pulmonary embolism or complications of necrosis of vital organs.

The most important points of treatment are:

(1) Exclude hypovolaemia by keeping the CVP between 14 and 18 mmHg and the PCWP between 15 and 20 mmHg.
(2) Exclude and treat right ventricular infarction (high CVP, tricuspid incompetence, ECG findings, scintigraphy, technetium pyrophosphate scan).
(3) Provide normal blood volume, give vasodilators and inotropics.
(4) Treat left ventricular failure with:
    (a) diuretics;
    (b) vasodilators, e.g. glyceryl trinitrate, sodium nitroprusside;
    (c) inotropics, e.g. dopamine, dobutamine, adrenaline;
    (d) intra-aortic balloon pump.
(5) Intracoronary streptokinase, RTPA (recombinant tissue plasminogen activator), PTCA or surgery.

The most common *arrhythmias* complicating myocardial infarction are:

(1) Ventricular fibrillation (see section on Cardiorespiratory arrest, p. 14).
(2) Ventricular ectopics. Correct hypoxia and hypokalaemia, then give lignocaine, 1 mg/kg/bolus followed by infusion of 30–60 µg/kg/min (average: 1–4 mg/min). If not effective switch to procainamide, 25 mg/min up to 1 g, with or without beta blockers (propranolol, 20 mg orally 6-hourly).
(3) Supraventricular tachycardia. If faster than 160/min and haemodynamic deterioration, perform DC cardioversion, followed by digoxin, 0.5–0.75 mg. If the patient is stable, i.v. verapamil may be an alternative as long as hypotension or low cardiac output are not present and the patient is not beta-blocked (5 mg over 2–5 min followed by the same dose in 5–10 min). Maintenance dose: digoxin, 0.25 mg/day; verapamil, 40–80 mg 8-hourly.
(4) Sinus bradycardia. Atropine, 0.5–1 mg i.v. followed by pacemaker if indicated (*see* section on Pacemakers, p. 22).

Heart block

In cases of anterior myocardial infarction with a new bundle branch block, a complete heart block may be anticipated. A pacemaker is indicated if some signs indicate imminent trifascicular block:

(a) right bundle branch block with left axis deviation and PR > 0.24 s;
(b) left bundle branch block and PR > 0.24 s;
(c) Möbitz type II block.

Obviously, when complete heart block is present, a pacemaker is mandatory.

Post-infarction ventricular arrhythmias

Post-infarction ventricular arrhythmias can be divided into two groups:

(a) early, starting with 24–48 h of the acute episode and caused by multiple transient substrates; and
(b) late, due to fixed anatomical areas in the border zone of the necrosis or aneurysm from islands of living myocardial cells, and likely to be recurrent.

The late ones are identifiable by mapping techniques and amenable to surgical attack when medical treatment is not effective.

The role of surgery is to interrupt or disengage a local arrhythmic circuit from the myocardium, while incurring minimal injury to the remaining heart. The surgical options are:

(a) coronary grafts alone;
(b) infarctectomy or aneurysmectomy;
(c) endocardial resection;
(d) encircling endocardial ventriculotomy;
(e) cryo-ablation.

Intra-operative mapping (activation, fragmentation) is necessary to localize the site of earliest activation in order to detect the arrhythmogenic focus and resect or disconnect it. Postoperative inotropic support, anticoagulation and predischarge electrophysiological study are important.

Ventricular aneurysm

Ventricular aneurysm is a localized ventricular wall protrusion with no contraction during the whole cardiac cycle and paradoxical movement. It can be diagnosed clinically by the presence of a diffuse precordial impulse, persistent ST elevation and a bulged cardiac silhouette, and confirmed by echo and radionuclide ventriculography.

The main complications associated with it are:

● arrhythmias
● embolism
● heart failure.

Once the treatment for ischaemic disease is complete (nitrates, beta blockers, calcium channel blockers) and associated arrhythmias are controlled, surgery may be recommended when persistent ventricular tachycardia refractory to medical treatment is present, or in cases of intractable heart failure, if the aneurysm is sufficiently circumscribed to be resectable. When the aneurysm involves massive areas of myocardium, transplantation is the best option.

Ventricular septal rupture

Ventricular septal rupture usually occurs during the first two weeks after the acute episode. The presence of a new systolic murmur and sudden deterioration suggests the diagnosis which is confirmed by

echo and cineangiography. The initial management is with inotropics, diuretics and intra-aortic balloon pump.

The most important controversy is the time of operation, as those
patients operated upon within the first two weeks have a high
mortality, probably due to the friability of the myocardium and the
severe clinical condition. When surgical treatment is decided upon,
patch closure of the defect is recommended, with or without
coronary grafts, depending on the angiography.

Acute mitral incompetence

Acute mitral incompetence following MI is clinically difficult to
differentiate from ventricular septal rupture. The diagnosis is clinically confirmed by echo and angiography. Treatment is combined
medical and surgical (mitral valve repair or replacement).

Abbreviations in cardiac medicine

Ao	aorta
AoV	aortic volume
BP	blood pressure
CI	cardiac index
CO	cardiac output
CVP	central venous pressure
EF	ejection fraction
HR	heart rate
IVC	inferior vena cava
LA	left atrium
LAP	left atrial pressure
LPA	left pulmonary artery
LV	left ventricle
LVEDP	left ventricular end diastolic pressure
LVOT	left ventricle outflow tract
LVSW	left ventricular systolic work
MAP	mean arterial pressure
MV	mitral valve
P	pulse
PA	pulmonary artery
PADP	pulmonary artery diastolic pressure
PASP	pulmonary artery systolic pressure
PAWP	pulmonary artery wedge pressure
PV	pulmonary valve
PVR	pulmonary vascular resistance

RA	right atrium
RAP	right atrial pressure
RPA	right pulmonary artery
RV	right ventricle
RVEDP	right ventricular end diastolic pressure
RVOT	right ventricle outflow tract
RVP	right ventricular pressure
RVSW	right ventricular systolic work
SI	stroke index; systolic index
SV	stroke volume; systolic volume
SVC	superior vena cava
SVR	systemic vascular resistance
SW	stroke work
TV	tricuspid valve

See also section on Cardiovascular formulae, p. 41.

Tables of normal values

Table 1.4 Normal cardiovascular pressures (mmHg)

PA	
Systolic	25 (15–30)
Diastolic	10 (5–15)
Mean	15 (10–20)
Wedge	10 (5–15)
LA	7 (4–12)
LV	
Systolic	120 (90–140)
End diastolic	7 (4–12)
RA	4 (0–8)
RV	
Systolic	25 (15–30)
End diastolic	4 (0–8)
Aorta	
Systolic	120 (90–140)
Diastolic	70 (60–90)
Mean	85 (70–105)
Blood pressure	
Systolic	90–140
Diastolic	60–90

Table 1.5 Left ventricular volumes

End diastolic volume (LVEDV)	70–85 ml/m²
End systolic volume (LVESV)	25–30 ml/m²
Systolic volume (LVSV)	45–55 ml/m²
Ejection fraction (EF) .	0.65–0.75 ml/m²
Stroke work (LVSW)	50–80 g/m/m²
Effective stroke volume	45–55 ml/m²
Regurgitant volume	Nil

Table 1.6 Distribution of cardiac output

Organ	Weight (kg)	Percentage body weight	Blood flow (ml/min)	Percentage cardiac output
Brain	1.4	2	775	15.0
Heart	0.3	0.43	175	3.3
Kidneys	0.3	0.43	1100	23.0
Liver	1.5	2.1	1400	29.0
Lungs	1.0	1.5	175	3.3
Muscles	27.8	39.7	1000	19.0
Rest	38.7	55.34	375	9.7

Table 1.7 Normal heart rate according to age

Age	Heart rate (beats/min)
< 1 month	120–190
1–6 months	110–180
6 months–1 year	100–170
1–3 years	90–160
3–6 years	80–150
6–15 years	70–140

Table 1.8 Average blood pressure according to age

Age	Blood pressure (mmHg)	
< 6 months	80/46	(MAP: 57)
6 months–1 year	89/60	(MAP: 70)
1–2 years	99/64	(MAP: 76)
2–4 years	100/65	(MAP: 77)
4–12 years	105/65	(MAP: 78)
12–15 years	118/68	(MAP: 85)
> 15 years	120/70	(MAP: 87)

Cardiovascular formulae

MAP (Mean arterial pressure)

$$= DP + \frac{SP - DP}{3}$$

Normal: 80–90 mmHg

CO (Cardiac output)

$$= Stroke\ volume \times Heart\ rate$$

Fick method:

$$= \frac{O_2\ consumption\ (ml/min)}{(A\text{–}V)\ O_2\ content\ (ml/l)} = \frac{V_{O_2}}{Ca_{O_2} - Cv_{O_2}}$$

Normal: 4–7 l/min

CI (Cardiac index)

$$= \frac{CO}{BSA}$$

Normal: 2.5–4.0 l/m^2

VR (Vascular resistance in general)

$$= \frac{Pressure}{Flow}$$

SVR (Systemic vascular resistance)

$$= \frac{MAP - CVP}{CO} \times 80$$

Normal: 1000–2000 dyne/cm^{-5}

PVR (Pulmonary vascular resistance)

$$= \frac{PAP - LAP}{CO} \times 80$$

Normal: 155–255 dyne/cm^{-5}

PCWP (Pulmonary capillary wedge pressure)

Measured by flotation catheter

Normal: 5–15 mmHg

PCP (Pulmonary capillary pressure)

$$= PCWP + 0.4 (PAP - PCWP)$$

Normal: 8–18 mmHg

SV (Stroke volume)

$$= LVEDV - LVESV$$

Normal: 50–60 ml

SI (Stroke index)

$$= \frac{SV}{BSA}$$

Normal: 35–40 ml/m^2

SW (Stroke work)

$$= SV \times MAP$$

Normal: 400–500 units

LVSW (Left ventricular stroke work)

$$= SV \times (MAP - PCWP) \times 0.136$$

Normal: 50–80 units

LVSW (from CO values)

$$= \frac{CO \times MAP \times 0.136}{HR}$$

RVSW (Right ventricular stroke work)

$$= \frac{CO \times MPAP \times 0.136}{HR}$$

Normal: 5–15 units

LVSWI (Left ventricular stroke work index)

$$= \frac{LVSW}{BSA}$$

Normal: 30–40

EF (Ejection fraction)

$$= \frac{LVEDV - LVESV}{LVEDV} \times 100$$

Normal: 65–75%

Oxygen delivery

$$= Ca_{O_2} \times CO \times 10$$

Normal: 1000 ml/min

$D(a–v)_{O_2}$ (Arteriovenous oxygen difference)

$$= (1.34 \times Hb) \times (Sa_{O_2} - Sv_{O_2})$$

Normal: 3.5–4.5 ml/100 ml

V_{O_2} (Oxygen consumption)

$$= D(a–v)_{O_2} \times CO \times 10$$

Normal: 250 ml/min

Oxygen utilization

$$= \frac{D(a–v)_{O_2}}{Ca_{O_2} \times CO}$$

Normal: Below 0.3

Ca_{O_2} (Arterial oxygen content)

$$= (Pa_{O_2} \times 0.0031) + (Hb \times 1.34 \times \% \text{ art. sat.})$$

Cv_{O_2} (Venous oxygen content)

$$= (Pv_{O_2} \times 0.0031) + (Hb \times 1.34 \times \% \text{ ven. sat.})$$

Cc_{O_2} (Alveolar blood oxygen content)

$$= (Pa_{O_2} \times 0.0031) + (Hb \times 1.34 \times 1)$$

Mixed venous oxygen content

$$= Ca_{O_2} - \frac{V_{O_2}}{CO}$$

Qs/Qt (physiologic shunt)

$$= \frac{Cc - Ca}{Cc - Cv} \times 100$$

Qp/Qs (Pulmonary to systemic flow ratio)

$$= \frac{\text{Systemic artery } S_{O_2} - \text{RA } S_{O_2}}{\text{LA } S_{O_2} - \text{PA } S_{O_2}}$$

$P_{A_{O_2}}$ (Oxygen alveolar pressure)

$$= [(\text{Bar press} - P_{H_2O}) \times F_{I_{O_2}}] - Pa_{CO_2}$$

$(A-a)D_{O_2}$ (Alveolo-arterial oxygen gradient)

$$= P_{A_{O_2}} - Pa_{O_2}$$

Qs/Qt from respiratory values

$$= \frac{\text{Unoxygenated cardiac output}}{\text{Total cardiac output}}$$

$$= \frac{(A-a)D_{O_2} \times 0.0031}{[(A-a)D_{O_2} \times 0.0031] + (Ca_{O_2} - Cv_{O_2})}$$

$$= \frac{(P_{A_{O_2}} - Pa_{O_2}) \times 0.0031}{[(P_{A_{O_2}} - Pa_{O_2}) \times 0.0031] + (Ca_{O_2} - Cv_{O_2})}$$

Body surface nomograms

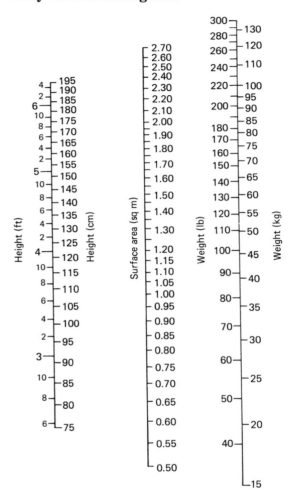

Figure 1.13 Body surface nomogram for total body perfusion for surface area, adults. To estimate the surface area of the patient, lay a straight edge across the figures for the patient's height and weight. Read the surface area at the point intersected by the straight edge

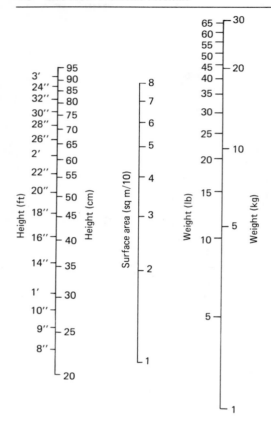

Figure 1.14 Body surface nomogram for total body perfusion for surface area, infants and children. To estimate the surface area of the patient, lay a straight edge across the figures for the patient's height and weight. Read surface area at the point intersected by the straight edge

Section II.

Cardiac Surgery

Intra-operative treatment

Junior staff should be present during induction of anaesthesia to help with speeding up one of the most critical periods of treatment. Once the anaesthetist has control of respiration, the Registrar should insert a urinary catheter and do whatever he can to help monitoring and intravenous cannulation.

Radial artery percutaneous cannulation should be preceded by confirmation of good collateral perfusion in the hand. If the radial stab fails, a very small cut-down rescues the situation and that of a haematoma forming after unsuccessful radial stabs. Other alternatives are the femoral or the brachial arteries. Central venous lines can be inserted in the internal jugular, subclavian, femoral or cephalic veins. Flushing of lines is fraught with risk: clots or air bubbles may reach the systemic circulation if put into venous lines when there is a right-to-left shunt; poor aseptic technique may infect valve prostheses through left atrial cannulae.

The period preliminary to bypass is a most hazardous one, as the patient still has the haemodynamic disorder and has to risk the reduction of his compensatory mechanisms by anaesthesia. The conditions of severe aortic stenosis with failure, pulmonary embolism with angor animi, acute myocardial infarction with angina, advanced mitral disease with cardiac cachexia, are ones which may require the setting up of supportive bypass or at least preparations completed for it before the induction of anaesthesia. The common femoral vessels can quickly and painlessly be exposed and taped under local anaesthesia. However, the combination of anaesthesia and adrenergic agents by skilled anaesthetists makes much of this preparation unnecessary.

Arrhythmias in the pre-open stage of the operation or in the poststernal closure stage may be very difficult to manage without reopening or desterilizing the field unless stick-on external defibrillator paddles are routinely used; these should always be affixed when reoperating on anyone as adhesions round the heart make the

47

application of internal paddles slow and traumatic, and it is in these patients that speed and the minimum of dissection are desirable.

On cardiopulmonary bypass oxygenation and systemic perfusion are maintained while the cardiac surgical procedure is being performed. Heparin prevents clotting when the blood contacts the 'external' circuits The blood is drained through cannulae in the cavae to the bypass machine, oxygenated and pumped back via the aortic cannula. Oxygenators can be of bubble or membrane type. The latter may be divided into parallel plate type, spiral coil type and hollow fibre membrane oxygenators.

Throughout the operation blood gases, electrolytes, blood glucose and clotting studies are measured. It is agreed that low-prime oxygenators primed with non-autologous blood provide the best conditions for the tissues, and that foreign blood may prejudice matters; some blood may be removed and the circulation replenished with Hartmann's solution during the pre-pump phase of the operation. The blood is available as a valuable autogenous fresh blood transfusion after the operation.

The preoccupations around the period of bypass are maintaining a good circulation to or protection of brain and heart, the avoidance of air embolus, and the provision of conditions that permit accurate and expeditious correction of the cardiac disorder. The last of these requirements often means that the heart must be without circulation; cold in various applications is used to protect its cells. The simplest is the irrigation of the contents of the pericardium with saline at low temperature (4 °C). Cardioplegia with St Thomas' solution at similar low temperatures permits 60–90 min without significant myocardial damage if the heart is kept below 20 °C.

Air ejection from heart into circulation is largely avoided by clamping the aorta, and when it is unclamped ensuring that the heart cannot eject by fibrillating it. When it is about to eject, all air must be excluded from all cardiac chambers and the aortic root by venting, continuous drainage, aspiration, hyperinflation of the lungs and turning the heart into various positions to allow the air to rise to the site whence it is removed.

When the operation is finished ventilation is resumed; the venous return is reduced first and the arterial flow decreased progressively in order to allow the heart to take over the circulation again. Once the patient is off bypass the cannulation lines are removed and protamine is given to neutralize heparin.

As bypass is concluded the heart may need stimulation with adrenergic agents and calcium. Sinus rhythm or atrial paced rhythm is important, and the maintenance of an adequate filling pressure for the ventricles ensured by monitoring both atrial pressures using lines left for this purpose postoperatively.

The intracardiac incisions should be adequately dry before the bypass is disconnected and the heparin reversed, and bleeding should be minimal before closure is commenced. Adequate drainage should always be provided. Care should be taken if the pericardium is closed as sick hearts may tolerate this pressure poorly. Rock-firm sternal closure prevents movement, pain and infection.

Transfer of patients from the table to intensive care is one of the most hazardous phases of the operation as the patient is not fully monitored, and there are disturbances of the haemodynamics from the inertial effects of movement and those of posture. There should thus be careful preparation of the bed-bay in intensive care, the route from theatre to it, and the bed brought into theatre to receive the patient.

All the bottle hangers, gas bottles, transducer-holders, bedclothes, pillows, dripstands, syringe pumps and portable defibrillator should be poised as the in-theatre connections are about to be undone. The pacemaker wires emerging from the patient should be carefully labelled and the pacemaker attached to appropriate ones if there is any likelihood whatsoever that pacing may need to be done *en route*. The balloon counterpulsation machine, if in action, will run without mains supply for a short time, but not long, and should be disconnected last in theatre and reconnected first in the unit, followed closely by syringe pumps which contain inotropic agents.

Postoperative management

Recovery from open heart surgery is done in an intensive care unit which should have as many of the following features as possible:

(1) Staffing should include:
   (a) 24 h-a-day medical cover on site capable of handling any likely emergency including pericardial tamponade, massive bleeding or the necessity for balloon counterpulsation;
   (b) a director of the unit who has charge of the patients while there without losing the available support from all other specialists involved in their management;
   (c) nursing staff capable of providing a 1:1 nurse:patient ratio including meal breaks, off-duty rotas, vacations, etc.;
   (d) 24 h availability of physiotherapists, radiographers and laboratory technicians.

(2) In addition to the normal ward duty rooms and offices, the architecture should allow for:
    (a) 'clean' and 'dirty' sides, space for at least 4% of the hospital patients' population, ventilation with air filtration, high volume to the 'very clean' area and pressure gradients from there to the 'very dirty' area and thence outdoors;
    (b) piped oxygen, air, suction and nitrous oxide, and adequate strategically placed power points including heavy duty ones for X-ray machines;
    (c) doctor's room with bed, bath and WC;
    (d) visitor's room;
    (e) a basic laboratory;
    (f) minor operations room;
    (g) rest room with snack-making facilities;
    (h) mini work shop.

Whether the ITU should be central, fully staffed, coping with all demands including coronary, neonatal, renal, respiratory, cardiovascular, general surgical and trauma, or the highly desirable concentration of expertise should be fragmented, is a question for the locals to decide, largely on a basis of numerical demands.

Monitoring

Central venous pressure

Central venous pressure (CVP) is a measure of right atrial pressure, primarily related to changes in the right ventricular system and secondarily to the function of the left side of the heart. It is useful particularly for monitoring intravascular volume. It can be measured by a catheter advanced from a peripheral vein to the SVC, IVC or right atrium. The most common veins used for it are the medial basilic, internal jugular, subclavian and femoral.

CVP can be measured in centimetres of water (cmH_2O) or in millimetres of mercury (mmHg). The conversion factors are:

$1 \, mmHg = 13.6 \, mmH_2O = 1.36 \, cmH_2O$
$1 \, cmH_2O = 1/1.36 \, mmHg.$

CVP is elevated in any situation that affects the right heart volumes and pressures, such as right ventricular failure, tricuspid valve disease, constrictive pericarditis, left ventricular failure and fluid overload.

When the CVP catheter is connected to an oscilloscope, the venous waves can be appreciated as:

'A' wave: reflects the atrial contraction and corresponds to the PR interval of the ECG. It precedes the arterial pulsation and the first cardiac sound. It is not present in cases of atrial fibrillation.

'C' wave: this is not always seen and corresponds with the RS–T junction of the ECG. It reflects the tricuspid valve closure at the beginning of ventricular systole.

'V' wave: this is secondary to the raised atrial pressure of ventricular systole.

There are also two deflections: 'X' (descendant aspect of 'A' wave) and 'Y' (descendant aspect of 'V' wave).

In some clinical situations these waves change in rather typical ways. For example, in constrictive pericarditis there are very prominent 'A' and 'V' waves that increase during inspiration. In atrioventricular dissociation (AV block, ventricular pacing and junctional rhythmus) there is lack of coordination between atrial and ventricular systole leading to atrial contraction at the time of ventricular systole against a closing tricuspid valve (i.e. simultaneous 'A' and 'C' waves – 'cannon' waves).

Electrocardiographic (ECG) monitoring

ECG monitoring is important for the early detection of potentially harmful arrhythmias. It is assumed that the patient has daily 12-lead ECGs. If any abnormal condition is detected in the monitor a new complete ECG must be taken.

Arrhythmias detected by ECG monitoring are:

- atrial ectopics
- supraventricular tachycardia
- atrial fibrillation
- atrial flutter
- nodal rhythm
- ventricular extrasystoles
- ventricular tachycardia
- ventricular fibrillation.

Bradycardias and heart blocks are also detected by ECG.

It is fallacious to diagnose acute ischaemia by the monitor only, and when it is suspected a full ECG must be performed.

Blood pressure monitoring

Blood pressure can be measured indirectly from inflating cuffs, by detecting the Korotkoff sounds, by cuff pressure oscillation or by blood vessel movements. Direct reading may be performed by using transducers. For this, a suitable artery (radial, brachial, femoral) is cannulated and connected to a transducer. Blood, air bubbles and foreign material must be avoided within the cuvette of the transducer or the catheter. The reference point is the heart level.

The systolic wave form reflects the stroke volume, aortic valve patency, the rate of ventricular contraction and the aortic wall compliance. The diastolic pressure reflects heart rate, peripheral vascular resistance and aortic valve competence. The normal arterial wave has an ascendant component, a notch and a descendant line. The notch reflects the closure of the aortic valve.

In aortic stenosis there is a slow and depressed peak upstroke. In aortic regurgitation there is large pulse pressure and low end diastolic pressure.

In hypovolaemia the trace oscillates with ventilation, and in it and left ventricular failure the area under the curve of the trace is small and sharp peaked.

Cardiac tamponade shows 'pulsus paradoxus', which is an exaggeration of the normal expiration rise/inspiration fall in blood pressure.

The arterial trace must be checked for damping, which may be due to a thrombus, air in the line or transducer, bad position of the arm or catheter bending. A dampened arterial waveform appears as a flattened version of the normal trace and the pressure will read low on the monitor. A falsely high reading may be due to overspiking when too wide bores are used, or air in the line or electronic mismatch permits oscillation.

Cardiac output

Cardiac output is sometimes very difficult to assess clinically in critically ill patients with complex cardiorespiratory problems and extensive operations. Pulmonary flotation catheters help to dictate appropriate therapy. The right ventricular wave pressure is recorded first. It has various phases according to the ventricular cycle – isometric contraction, ejection phase, diastole and diastasis.

The right ventricular end-diastolic pressure is elevated in cases of pulmonary hypertension, pulmonary stenosis, right ventricular failure, pericarditis and ventricular septal defect.

The catheter is advanced to the pulmonary artery and its systolic, diastolic and mean pressures are confirmed. These are elevated in cases of increased pulmonary blood flow, pulmonary hypertension (primary or secondary) and left ventricular failure. In patients with normal lungs and normal mitral valve the PA pressure is an indicator of left ventricular end-diastolic pressure (LVEDP). The higher the LVEDP, the stiffer or fuller the ventricle.

The wedge pressure is obtained by inflating the balloon at the end of the catheter which then occludes a peripheral branch of the pulmonary artery. Over-inflation may cause damage of the endothelium of the pulmonary artery. Also, if the balloon is not deflated, pulmonary infarction may be caused. The wedge pressure reflects the left atrial pressure with a characteristic shape made by an 'A' wave (left atrial systole), a 'C' wave (closure of the atrioventricular valve), and a 'V' wave (bulging of the valve into the atrium in systole). The wedge is elevated in left ventricular failure, fluid overload and mitral valve disease. There are huge 'V' waves in acute mitral incompetence, large right-to-left shunts, and in severe coronary artery disease.

Cardiac output is measured by injecting a sterile solution, cooler than the body temperature, into the catheter sited in the pulmonary artery from side holes upstream from the catheter tip temperature transducer, and calculating flow by thermodilution.

Some complications associated with flotation catheters are thrombophlebitis, ventricular irritability and pulmonary haemorrhage.

Postoperative cardiac care

The basic observations after heart surgery must include:

(1) General condition: peripheral circulation, distress, bleeding, conscious level, movements, chest inspection.
(2) Drainage rate through mediastinal drains.
(3) ECG monitoring: rate, rhythm, QRS/ST patterns, pacing wires connected appropriately.
(4) Mean arterial pressure around 75–85 mmHg.
(5) Central venous pressure around 10–15 mmHg.
(6) Left atrial pressure around 15–23 mmHg.
(7) Urine output about 0.5–1.0 ml/kg/h.
(8) Fluids and electrolytes: 1.0–2.0 ml/kg/h of iso-osmolar solution. Potassium to be kept between 4.0 and 4.5 mmol/l.
(9) Ventilations: V_T of 10–15 ml/kg; IMV: 8–12/min.
(10) Blood balance.
(11) Blood gases.
(12) Chest X-rays.
(13) Nursing care: pressure points, mucous membranes, etc.
(14) Physiotherapy and respiratory therapy.

General care of the cardiovascular system

Fundamental to the maintenance of life is the supply of necessities to every cell in the body. There must be enough blood of the right constitution propelled to every cell at the right speed and at the right temperature. Failure of any of these requirements will soon show by various reflexes and later by evidence of metabolic derangement. Ideally even the reflex evidence should not be allowed to appear. The reflex manifestations of cell deprivation of anything include the feeling of dyspnoea which may result in 'fighting' the ventilator, vasoconstriction which may itself worsen the cells' supply failure, sweating, reduced urinary output, anxiety, and tachycardia (late in infants – bradycardia). The late metabolic manifestations include acidosis, hyperkalaemia, falling mixed venous oxygen saturation and arterial saturation and the effects of deprivation on essential organs like the liver, kidneys and brain.

The supply failure involving the composition of the blood most commonly is a deficiency of oxygen (supply, carrying power or availability). Other nutrients include glucose (and a means of making it available, i.e. insulin) and the precursors of metabolic enzymes such as vitamins.

The delivery of the blood is the task of the cardiovascular system. There must be enough blood to fill the vessels and to give the ventricles enough filling pressure to prime them fully. The normal blood volume is 7% of the body weight or 3 l/sq m. A fall below this would cause reflex vasoconstriction and tachycardia initially, with metabolic changes if hypovolaemia is not corrected. When more than 10% of the intravascular volume is lost the clinical manifestations of hypovolaemia are present. This is true in children as well.

Hypovolaemia

The hypovolaemic patient is hypotensive, hypoperfused, tachycardic, with collapsed neck veins, weak pulses and small urine output.

The most important causes of hypovolaemia in the cardiac postoperative patient are:

(1) *Bleeding.* As stated on p. 57, the presence of more than 200 ml/h in the thoracic drains for four consecutive hours, or more than 400 ml at any time, generally demands re-opening. Sometimes the cause of bleeding is in one of the multiple holes the surgeon has to make (aortic cannulation, aortic cardioplegia, atrial cannulation, cardiotomies, ventricular or pulmonary artery vents, coronary anastomosis, etc.). On the other hand, defective

clotting factors may be responsible. The adequacy of heparin reversal affects the accelerated clotting time (ACT), which can be cellite or saline. Abnormalities of the coagulation tests should be corrected by administration of specific factors (e.g. protamine, platelets, fresh frozen plasma or whole blood).

(2) *Other causes.* These include, in particular, water loss and/or excessive vasodilatation. The choice of volume for replacement depends on the cause and the packed cell volume (PCV). Blood or plasma expanders should be used to arrive at a PCV of around 35%.

Hypervolaemia

The other extreme of the spectrum is hypervolaemia. A rise above the normal limits can easily cause congestive cardiac failure, with oedema of whichever part of the body is congested (usually the lungs first, as the left heart normally fails first).

The pressure in the veins and left atrium are guides to the adequacy of the blood volume and normally parallel each other, but sometimes the right or left heart fails alone, and if the latter, filling a patient up until he has a normal right heart filling pressure may elevate the left filling pressure to the level producing pulmonary oedema. In these uncommon situations, therefore, left atrial pressure is invaluable but technically difficult to obtain unless a tube has been left at operation. However, Swan-Ganz catheterization provides pulmonary wedge pressure, or the pulmonary artery end-diastolic pressure from a floated-in catheter can be used as a left heart filling pressure if there is not active pulmonary hypertension (in which circumstances the right sided pressure would be the critical one anyway).

Once a good output and normally filled peripheral veins demonstrate normovolaemia, the filling pressures may be allowed to fall to levels which reflect the excellence of the heart. The maximum permissible pressures depend somewhat on the integrity of the semipermeability of the capillaries, in that after a poor perfusion oedema may develop in tissues at much lower capillary pressures than normally. The same will be seen if the plasma colloid osmotic pressure is reduced by hypoalbuminaemia. Normally, however, right sided pressures of 15 mmHg and left sided ones of 24 mmHg should not be exceeded, unless seen in hypovolaemia plus vasoconstriction, when vasodilators will help to resolve the problem.

In the presence of a normal volume of normally composed blood, tissue malperfusion is the result of heart failure. This in turn may be due to haemodynamic, arrhythmic or myocardial disorder, and the myocardium may be afflicted by cellular damage or vascular insufficiency. The distinction is usually obvious clinically, and if a remediable 'plumbing' problem underlies the heart failure, no time should be lost in correcting it surgically, especially if its remedy is simple as in the case of postoperative tamponade from blood. An arrhythmic problem is usually immediately apparent and capable of solution.

Myocardial insufficiency

Postoperative non-ischaemic myocardial insufficiency is the most common and least welcome of all the causes of postoperative cardiac failure. It may be the result of prolonged operative ischaemia with inadequate myocardial protection, air in the coronary vessels, damage to coronaries by cannulae, part of a generalized body insult from prolonged cardiopulmonary bypass ('total body confusion') with pump oxygenator systems of high damage potential rather than newer disposable clear-fluid-prime membrane or bubble oxygenators and accurate roller or pulsatile pumps. It is characterized by low fixed stroke volume, low diastolic compliance, and slow contraction velocity (a stiff ventricle).

Although inotropic agents may speed up and strengthen myocardial contraction, they may make an already spastic ventricle even more so, especially if it is already hypertrophic as in severe aortic stenosis, when the large muscle mass relative to coronary supply may complete the prerequisites for subendocardial necrosis. As high a filling pressure as the capillary permeability will stand (pulmonary oedema shows promptly by increased alveolar–arterial Po_2 gradient), and a peripheral dilator like glyceryl trinitrate or sodium nitroprusside to reduce ventricular workload are at least as important as catecholamines in the management of this problem. Correction of acidosis, hyperkalaemia, arrhythmias and anoxia are essential preliminary measures. If all these moves fail, balloon counterpulsation will augment cardiac output considerably.

Ischaemic myocardial insufficiency is not often seen after open heart operations but is a common sight in coronary care units. Management is the same as for the non-ischaemic variety but glucose-insulin-potassium may have a place, with anti-arrhythmics, of higher importance. The fundamental cause of the problem – blocked coronary arteries – may be a surgical problem even at this late stage, if a large amount of ischaemia surrounds the infarction, or the coronary blocks during coronary angiography or angioplasty on the threshold of theatre.

Haemodynamic problems

Haemodynamic causes of postoperative cardiac failure include tamponade, which shows by falling output, rising pulse and venous pressures, excessive 'pulsus paradoxus', Kussmaul venous sign, and a marked fall in pressures with isoprenaline rather than the improvement seen when myocardial failure underlies the low output.

Re-opening in ITU

Postoperative cardiac tamponade is notoriously difficult to identify, though will never be found if not contemplated. Even ultrasound is not a completely reliable way of excluding this problem and re-opening may be the only way to do so. Bleeding of over 200 ml/h, not diminishing or increasing, is an indication for re-opening but, in

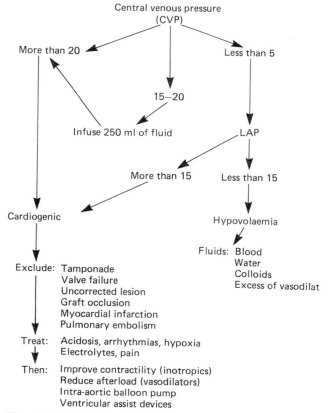

Figure 2.1 Scheme for diagnosis and treatment of low cardiac output syndrome after cardiac surgery

this context and in that of deliberately exploring for tamponade, the facilities of the theatre should be used. Massive bleeding, or the deterioration of the heart to a lethal degree without adequate explanation justify re-opening of the sternotomy in ITU. Experience has shown that this resource has not resulted in more wound infection provided the usual standards of asepsis normal in theatre are applied in the unit. Sterile thoracotomy packs are available and proper scrub and gown measures can usually be followed. It is important for those planning the equipment to ensure that the packs include wire-cutters for sternotomy wires and that the suction available is strong enough to evacuate big clots.

In summary, if the heart is not furnishing enough output, management should check that:

- there is not a surgically correctable lesion;
- the blood volume, gases, acid-base status is correct;
- no correctable or controllable arrhythmias exist;

and then stimulating the ventricle with calcium, catecholamines, atrial pacing, and reduce the ventricular workload with peripheral vasodilators.

Although it is not ideal to treat patients according to rigid rules and tables, a general guide helps to define and remember some important points of diagnosis and treatment. The scheme shown in Figure 2.1 is just one of these guidelines.

Inotropics used in intensive care

Table 2.1 Inotropics used in intensive care

	Adrenaline	Noradrenaline	Isoprenaline	Dopamine	Dobutamine	Salbutamol
Vasoconstriction	+ + +	+ + + +	0	0 to + + +	+	0
Vasodilatation	+	0	+ + + +	+ +	+	+ + + +
Renal dilatation	0	0	0	+ + + +	0	0
Rate increase	+ + + +	+ + + +	+ + + +	+ + +	+	+ + +
Contractility	+ + + +	+ + + +	+ + + +	+ + + +	+ + + +	0
Arrhythmias	+ + + +	+ + + +	+ + + +	+ +	+	+
Preload	Variable	Increased	Decreased	Variable	Variable	Variable
Afterload	Variable	Increased	Decreased	Variable	Variable	Variable

Note: Alpha effect is vasoconstriction.
          Beta-2 effect is vasodilatation.
          Beta-1 effect is heart contractility, rate and conduction.
          Delta effect is renal vasodilatation.

Formulae

(1) *For adrenaline, noradrenaline and isoprenaline*:
   (BW in kg × 3)/100 = mg to add to 50 ml of solution
   Then: 1 ml/h = 0.01 µg/kg/min
   Range: 2–20 ml/h
(2) *For dopamine and dobutamine*:
   (BW in kg × 3) = mg to add to 50 ml solution
   Then: 1 ml/h = 1 µg/kg/min
   Range: 2–20 ml/h

Doses of main inotropics

Table 2.2 Doses of inotropic drugs

Drug	Dose (µg/kg/min)	Dose (µg/h)	Dilution	Speed range (ml/h)
Adrenaline	0.02–0.2	72–1280	1 mg/100 ml (10 µg/ml)	7–120
Noradrenaline	0.01–0.2	36–1280	1 mg/100 ml (10 µg/ml)	4–120
Isoprenaline	0.02–0.2	72–1280	1 mg/100 ml (10 µg/ml)	7–120
Dopamine	2–20	7–128 mg/h	200 mg/100 ml (2 mg/ml)	3–60
Dobutamine	2–20	7–128 mg/h	250 mg/ml) (2.5 mg/ml)	3–50
Salbutamol	0.02–0.2	72–1280	1 mg/100 ml (10 µg/ml)	7–120

Note: If it is necessary to restrict the amount of fluids, then double the doses or halve the diluent.

Speed range of inotropic drugs when drug strength changes

Table 2.3 Speed range (in ml/h) when drug strength changes

	1 mg/100 ml	*2 mg/100 ml*	*4 mg/100 ml*	*8 mg/100 ml*
Adrenaline Noradrenaline Isoprenaline Salbutamol	7–120	3–60	2–30	1–15

Vasodilators used in postoperative cardiac surgery

Table 2.4 Vasodilators used in postoperative cardiac surgery

Drug	Artery	Vein	Onset (min)	Duration	Dose
Nitroprusside	+	+	1	2–5 min	0.3–15.0 µg/kg/min
Nitroglycerine	–	+	1–2	10 min	0.3–4.0 µg/kg/min
Diazoxide	+	–	1	4–12 h	300 mg i.v. up to 3 times
Trimetaphan	+	–	1	2–5 min	1–15 mg/min
Hydralazine	+	–	10–20	2–6 h	5–20 mg i.v.
Phentolamine	+	–	1–2	20 min	0.1–2.0 mg/min, up to 60 mg

Formula

For sodium nitroprusside
   (BW in kg × 3)/10 = mg to add to 50 ml of solution

Then: 1 ml/h = 0.1 µg/kg/min
Range: 1–15 ml/h

The intra-aortic balloon

The general principle of the intra-aortic balloon pump (IABP) is to evacuate the stroke volume from the aorta in systole, thus making room for the effortless ejection of that volume by the ventricle, and then in diastole to replace this volume in the aorta after aortic valve closure, thus doing work against pressure and boosting diastolic pressure with particular benefit to the predominantly diastolic coronary flow.

Access to the arterial system is obtained by the smallest possible 'invasion' by a thin catheter with a 50 ml balloon at its terminal 10 cm. The balloon is located in the descending aorta from the subclavian down to the supradiaphragmatic aorta. A low density, low viscosity gas such as helium permits more rapid and complete balloon excursion, but carbon dioxide is less risky if the balloon leaks. The balloon excursions are monitored either by having an external 'master' balloon connected to the working 'slave' balloon, or by means of monitoring systems within the drive unit. The drive unit is triggered by the QRS complex of the ECG and the clinician can set the delay between this and the deflation of the balloon, the duration of the deflation and the subsequent reflation.

The ideal is obviously for the balloon to deflate as ventricular systole generates pressure equal to the aortic pressure and to reflate at the moment the aortic valve closes. In practice, the arterial trace is watched and the balloon timing moved to achieve a maximal diastolic 'balloon wave'.

Cardiac energy is spared, the coronary blood flow is increased and systemic perfusion improves from decreased myocardial oxygen consumption, increased cardiac output, and reduced pulmonary congestion, diminishing left-to-right shunts and improving aerobic metabolism.

General indications for the IABP are:
- cardiogenic shock secondary to myocardial infarction
- unstable angina with deteriorating condition
- intractable arrhythmias in coronary patients
- acute ventricular septal rupture
- acute mitral valve incompetence
- septic shock
- haemodynamically unstable general surgical patients
- post-cardiopulmonary bypass heart failure
- intraoperative myocardial infarction
- any case of severe low cardiac output.

From the point of view of numbers:
- cardiac index below 1.8 ml/min/m²
- ejection fraction less than 20%
- LVEDP above 20 mmHg

Some contraindications for its use are:
- aortic valve incompetence
- dissecting aortic aneurysm
- relatively advanced peripheral vascular disease

Some reported complications are:
- aortic dissection
- atheromatous plaque embolism
- femoral artery obstruction
- infection
- haemorrhage

Heparin is used while the balloon is in at 30 units/kg loading dose, and 500–1000 units 2-hourly to keep cellite ACT between 150 and 200.

The respiratory system in cardiac surgery

The lungs of the average cardiac surgical patient are rarely normal, having been exposed to congestive heart failure, high flow rates from left-to-right shunts, the development of large bronchial collaterals in cyanotic conditions, and even to tobacco-induced bronchitis in the coronary patients. Not only may the pulmonary vascular resistance be raised, but also the airway resistance from bronchial venous congestion or smoke inhalation.

Operation – especially long bypass with non-autologous blood primes and imperfect management of pumping – increases the lung water content and introduces diffusion defects, and manipulation of the lung at surgery, trauma to the airways, irritation with inhalation anaesthesia, retained secretions and areas of atelectasis resulting from ineffective coughing from pain/sedation combined with totally absorbed inhaled gases, all make their contribution to a mixed respiratory insufficiency.

Available data for respiratory evaluation consist of the appearance and respiratory activity of the patient, his blood gas levels, the content and pressure of the inhaled gases, and the volumes exhaled by the patient, which could be analysed for content though not done at present routinely. The inhaled gases can be varied widely in fully sedated patients on respirators and the consequences observed. In patients ventilating spontaneously the arterial Po_2 relative to the inhaled Po_2 is a guide to the existence of diffusion abnormalities or the presence of shunting in the lung, and the Po_2 is a guide to ventilation-perfusion defects, but artificial ventilation sometimes obscures the latter correlations.

The response of the alveolar–arterial gradient to a brisk diuresis is a way of distinguishing shunting (no response) from alveolar oedema with diffusion defect (improvement), and conversely the response of the gradient to physiotherapy or bag-squeezing is favourable in the atelectatic shunting cases.

Artificial ventilation is frequently applied after open-heart operations for the first postoperative night to allow the cardiovascular status to steady up, and as a part of the 'maximum care' philosophy. Its use is indicated for failure of respiratory drive, the inadequacy of ventilatory strength, and intubation at least is required for failure of coughing and when a positive pressure must be applied to the airways in the absence of an oral or nasal means of achieving this. All ventilation techniques are designed to increase lung volumes and minimize intrapulmonary shunt. The means of delivery of ventilation is a tube of non-irritating material passed through the nose or (less satisfactory) the mouth; tracheostomy is more likely to be associated with mediastinal infection and is no longer necessary for the prevention of vocal cord abrasion since the modern tubes are well tolerated for many days.

The ventilator should be matched to the patient's requirements. Patients with low or changing pulmonary compliance should have a volume-cycled respirator which will ventilate the same amount regardless of the pressures it generates to achieve it; where there is a leak in the airway – which may be intentional as a loose leaky tube does less damage especially in babies – then a pressure-cycled respirator is best; when a patient needs help rather than complete control of ventilation, a ventilator which he can trigger is best since the respiratory reflexes are more ideal than the regulation of a machine by a number of delayed and fallible blood estimations.

The expired gas should be monitored in all cases with an 'alarm' monitor. After operation in babies spontaneous ventilation with constant positive airways pressure (CPAP) is better than artificial ventilation. Patients with pulmonary oedema are helped by maintaining a positive end expiratory pressure (PEEP) with positive pressure ventilation.

Safe weaning from ventilation may be done by leaving the patient to breathe spontaneously (with or without CPAP) but an ever-diminishing baseline of intermittent mandatory ventilation (IMV) must also be applied to keep him from fatal underventilation.

At all times when normal nasal humidification channels are bypassed the inhaled gases should be fully humidified. All ventilation apparatus should be fully sterilized between uses, and aseptic techniques should be used for all intra-airway procedures. Wherever there is total dependence on a ventilator, full 'alarm' systems should exist for the supply of gases, heat and humidification of inspired gases and the volume of expired gas (see also p. 120 and Table 4.3).

Once committed to ventilation, the habitual reluctance to give large doses of analgesics for fear of lowering ventilation drive need apply no longer, and truly analgesic concentrations can be achieved with benefit to the tolerance of the tube and ventilator as well as peripheral circulation and general well-being. Though the poppy derivatives are good, additional cooperation can be wrought from the patient with sedatives like diazepam, and only in the rare circumstance (when it is highly likely that there is something serious wrong like blood loss or tamponade) has one to resort to curarizing the respirator 'victim' (when it is preferable to use vercuronium rather than curare as the latter may cause peripheral vascular collapse and abdominal distension).

Excessive levels of oxygen may harm the lung, and the proportion of oxygen in the inspired air should not exceed that necessary to achieve Pao_2 of 100–120 mmHg (12–15 kPa).

Far-reaching biochemical disturbances result from over-ventilation to the point of lowering the $Paco_2$, and a slightly higher than normal $Paco_2$ is tolerated by a well sedated patient and is safer and even beneficial in terms of increased peripheral perfusion and cardiac output. If a large tidal volume as well as high inspired Po_2 is necessary to maintain a satisfactory Pao_2, with the possible consequence of lowering the $Paco_2$, a piece of tube can be added to the connection to the airway tube to increase the dead space.

After correction of large left-to-right shunts, the lungs may continue to be oedematous and non-compliant for some time and require both increased airway pressures to relieve oedema and mechanical assistance to move the stiff lungs. Previously oligaemic lungs may become oedematous when full circulation is restored, especially if arterial collaterals from the aorta have not been tied off at the time of corrective operation. Pulmonary hypertension of an active type may reduce pulmonary perfusion relative to ventilation, reduce cardiac output due to right heart inadequacy and also is frequently associated with excessive secretions.

Discontinuation of ventilator

Discontinuing ventilatory assistance may be carried out when the patient looks well, without cardiovascular problem, the airway is clear, respiratory movements uninhibited, and Pao_2 is > 300 mmHg (40 kPa) on 100% inspired oxygen. Then a trial of ventilation with a T-tube carrying humidified oxygen–air mixture in the proportion achievable with a face mask (60%) is justified. If then the tidal air is good (over 10 ml/kg), the respiratory rate is below 30/min, the patient is not restless, sweating, dyspnoeic or moving his alae nasae, and $Paco_2$ is < 50 mmHg (6.5 kPa) and stable, then the tube can be removed. This should be done at the beginning of the working day, when continued evaluation and re-intubation can be done without waiting for off-duty staff. A reasonable timetable for routine postoperative patients ventilated on the first postoperative night is as follows:

8.00–8.30 a.m.
    (assuming the patient is awake, cooperative, looks fit and has a clear chest): ventilate with 100% oxygen
8.30 a.m.: blood gas sample, put onto T-tube with 60% oxygen

9.00 a.m.: analyse gases. If the 8.30 Pa_{O_2} < 300 mmHg (40 kPa) the artificial ventilation should be resumed, improve cardiac status or relieve pulmonary oedema, congestion or obstruction. If the 9.00 Pco_2 > 55 mmHg (7 kPa), ventilation should be resumed until the patient is either more wakeful or strong enough to ventilate himself adequately.

Paediatric surgery

Unless mechanical assistance to shift the air is required, the best support to postoperative children is provided by CPAP, next best is spontaneous ventilation, then artificial ventilation with PEEP, and worst of all is artificial ventilation without PEEP, as judged by low cardiac output and blood gas levels.

The best intubation technique in babies is the Jackson-Rees nasal tube, and it is wise to have a fit in the trachea that is not too snug, so that damage to the subglottic area is minimized; when the airways pressure is always above atmospheric, secretions from the throat will not get past the tube as the air is blowing away. Allowance should be made for the leak when calculating tidal volume required from the paediatric ventilators. Full humidification is essential in children to prevent blockage of the tube.

Some normal volumes in children are:

- Tidal volume: 7 ml/kg (neonates: 6 ml/kg)
- Dead space: tidal volume × 0.3
- Respiratory rate: neonates 30/min; 1–13 years: 24 (age/2)/min
- Blood volume: 80 ml/kg (neonates: 100 ml/kg)

Calculation of the ventilation volumes should take into account the tubing of the ventilator and the dead space of the system, since the proportion of these relative to the tiny infant is so much more than in larger patients.

With high airway pressure, higher than normal minute volumes may be necessary and dead space may be needed to keep the Pa_{CO_2} from being reduced.

Discontinuation of ventilation in children may be done with intermittent mandatory ventilation, and continuous airway pressure is a great help. The presence of a small catheter to the bifurcation of the trachea enables a high airway pressure, high oxygen percentage, and repeated suction to be achieved with little interference, and should be more often employed, especially in neonates, during weaning from ventilation.

Therapeutic bronchoscopy

The accumulation of bronchial secretions may not always be able to be coughed up by the patient or sucked out of the mouth or pharynx by nursing or physiotherapy staff. A sucker can be introduced into the larynx and trachea either under vision or 'blind' and will stimulate coughing and remove the results to good effect. Secretions may be inspissated in the lower bronchial tree, or the patient too weak or poorly ventilated to bring even liquid secretions up from there. In these circumstances therapeutic bronchoscopy has to be done.

In a crashing emergency, which we try to avoid, the patient may be so black that there is no time to spare for anaesthesia, and anyway so far gone that it is not cruel to bronchoscope him without attempting anaesthesia. The ideal is a short general anaesthetic because it is total but without residual depression of movement or sensation, as well as being the most humane.

Local anaesthesia is acceptable in the absence of an anaesthetist. Intravenous diazepam is supplemented by sucking an anaesthetic lozenge after which cotton wool soaked in topical lignocaine is held on each pyriform fossa for 2 min, the throat is sprayed with topical lignocaine, then the cords are sprayed with it using a laryngoscope, and the bronchoscope is introduced through which the carina is sprayed, and the sucking out is performed.

If the procedure has to be done in the patient's bed with the patient conscious, it is best to stand on a stool above the patient's bedhead with the patient sitting up in his usual position. Once the bronchoscope is past the cords the patient is entirely at the mercy of the bronchoscopist and vigilance must be exercised not to be unnecessarily cruel.

Complications after coronary surgery

During diagnostic procedures (angiography), the main complications are related to the arteries used for access to the coronary system (brachial, femoral) which can bleed or become infected. Damage to the coronaries, either by catheter or by balloon angioplasty, makes surgery advisable should the patient show ECG changes, severe angina or haemodynamic impairment.

The main complication of coronary surgery is myocardial infarction, which can occur pre-operatively following abrupt change in or stopping of previous medications, or during operation due to poor myocardial protection or insufficient pressures during the procedure.

Surgical technical failure could be due to:
- inability to find the vessels
- incomplete opening of them
- inadequate distal flow to poor vessels
- incomplete endarterectomy
- occlusion of the artery by stitches
- kinking of the grafts
- inadequate venous length
- defective proximal anastomosis

After the operation the main problems are low cardiac output due to incomplete revascularization, myocardial damage, drug-induced depression and other causes outlined in Figure 2.1. If graft occlusion is suspected or if the patient's condition deteriorates rapidly, surgery is indicated if emergency previous angiography shows obstruction.

Any new ischaemic changes or patterns suggesting myocardial infarction should be examined thoroughly and complementary tests such as serial ECG, cardiac enzymes and radionuclide scanning as screening tests for the need for angiography may be performed.

Postoperative hypertension must be avoided after coronary grafts to minimize bleeding. Sodium nitroprusside, with or without labetalol infusions, is recommended.

Recurrent angina after previous bypass surgery should be studied carefully starting with an exercise test and, depending on it, angiography. If the distal vessels are poor or the ventricular function severely depleted the patient is treated pharmacologically; if distal vessels are good and a graft is stenosed, PTCA may be attempted; otherwise, surgery is indicated. In cases of re-operation for grafts, the femoral artery should be routinely exposed at the time of operation, not only to anticipate massive bleeding at the sternal re-opening, but also in case the aorta is too difficult to cannulate.

Fluids, electrolytes and the renal system after cardiac surgery

Fluid

Balance charts provide much occupational therapy for those producing them but, except in the critical few hours of intensive care, are of little practical value compared with regular scrupulous weighing. Metabolism of food produces up to a pint of water a day and insensible losses may lose this much. The food and the faeces vary in the amount of water contained and patients unconfined vary in their reliability. Fluid intake should be:

- 1 mg/kg/h in those over 20 kg
- 1.5 ml/kg/h in those between 10 and 20 kg
- 2 ml/kg/h in those under 10 kg

Increased initial allowance can be made for moderate dehydration with a dry mouth and bright eyes, which constitutes about 5% of the body weight in children, and severe dehydration with fast pulse, sunken eyes, scant urine and deep respiration, which constitutes about 10% of the weight in children. These deficiencies can be made up in the first 6 h.

Cardiac patients may have too much water on board in their extracellular space, where it will do no harm in the periphery; if in the lung, then severe pulmonary dysfunction results and urgent means like reduction of blood volume or afterload or rapid diuresis are required.

If correctly hydrated and with a normal circulation, 30 ml/h of urine should be forthcoming in the adult and a reduction below this suggests too little water, a poor circulation or some deficiency of renal function.

Electrolytes

Potassium

Potassium is the most immediately important of the electrolytes. Most patients with chronic valvular disease who have been on diuretics have a total body deficiency of up to one-third, and their tissues soak up the plasma potassium rapidly when a bounding circulation is restored, and at the same time much excess water may be eliminated carrying out more potassium. Thus it is the patients who have experienced the most haemodynamic benefit from surgery who are the most prone to get hypokalaemic and die of ventricular fibrillation. On the other hand, patients with a deteriorating cardiac action get rapidly worse as the resulting cellular acidosis and loss of potassium into the plasma further depress cardiac action.

The urine usually contains about 50 mEq/l, and this or the measured urinary potassium content should be restored to the patient who is having diuresis with frequent checks on the plasma level. Replacing urinary losses will also prevent the routine administration of potassium to a patient whose urinary output is falling as his cardiac action deteriorates and his plasma potassium level rises.

Some give 1 mEq of potassium per minute of bypass to patients who have been on diuretics (on the empirical assumption that the longer bypasses need more valves replaced and have probably been on the most diuretics), 10 ml 10% calcium chloride as bypass is ending, and then replace the urinary losses of potassium as they occur (e.g. 5 mEq KCl/100 ml of urine passed) plus a little to compensate for shift of potassium into cells (e.g. 10 mEq/50 g of glucose in the postoperative intravenous solution).

Magnesium

This is often significantly deficient after open heart surgery, which frequently mimics hypokalaemia, though results in a weaker cardiac contraction and may cause psychological disturbances. Prevention with 300 mg/day of magnesium chloride orally and up to 35 mg of magnesium as the sulphate per 500 ml of postoperative intravenous fluid, after using 120 mg of magnesium as the sulphate in the heart-lung machine, keeps the postoperative serum levels normal. Great care is necessary to avoid overload when renal function is depressed.

Calcium

There is a large reservoir in everyone's bones, but acute low levels of calcium may depress cardiac function, which is known to depend for contraction on calcium. Therefore, when large volumes of citrated blood are being given it is wise to give 3.5 ml of 10% calcium chloride slowly for each unit of blood used.

Sodium

Also essential for normal myocardial contraction, sodium is often deficient in patients who have been on diuretics, but caution is advised in heart failure as too much sodium will hold too much water in the patient and may worsen failure. One unit per day of one-fifth saline should fill the patient's need for sodium.

Renal failure

Less than 30 ml/h of urine in an adult should arouse suspicion; less than 20 ml/h is oliguria and less than 10 ml/h is renal failure. The circulation is confirmed as adequate before impugning the kidneys, and the patient is assumed not to be dehydrated. Escalating doses of frusemide are used, and it is now known that doses up to 1 g can be tolerated. Failure of this response helps to confirm renal failure.

Confirmed renal failure demands the reduction of all fluid to 500 ml/day, with which the day's calories should be given. Excess water can be eliminated by making the patient sweat so that dialysis can be delayed until the potassium or the urea levels demand it. The potassium can be kept low with ion exchange resins and by treating acidosis, and potassium can be temporarily lowered with a glucose–insulin mixture (100 ml of 50% dextrose with 10–20 units of insulin) and its cardiac effects alleviated with calcium chloride.

Peritoneal dialysis requires no anticoagulation, is easily managed in the average ITU, and provides calories in the glucose absorbed. If the renal failure persists beyond 10 days a renal biopsy should be obtained.

Acid-base disturbances

Acidosis is the most common acid-base disturbance, and if metabolic is the result of low cardiac output and lactic and pyruvic acid from the tissues. It worsens cardiac action further. Its treatment is the administration of sodium bicarbonate and sometimes tris-hydroxy-methyl-aminomethane (THAM) until the pH, bicarbonate and base excess are normal, plus the treatment of the predisposing circulatory insufficiency.

Metabolic alkalosis occurs in about half of really ill postoperative patients at some stage, often associated with abnormally large potassium losses. The replacement of chloride to correct the acidosis and hypokalaemia is important. Nasogastric aspirations should be discontinued as soon as possible, and hyperventilation avoided. Thiazide diuretics should be minimized, and osmotic diuretics such as mannitol may be preferred if necessary in these cases. Potassium chloride to stop urinary hydrogen ion loss is the basis of treatment.

Nutritional aspects of cardiac surgery

Malnutrition (inadequate provision of substrates for growth, activity and tissue repair) causes loss of cellular mass (muscular and visceral), malfunction of vital organs, abnormal polymorphonuclear chemotaxis, dropping in the number of T cell rosettes, intracellular contraction, extracellular expansion and increased susceptibility to infection and delayed wound healing as well as higher incidence of respiratory failure secondary to muscular wasting.

The heart is, of course, affected by malnutrition, with deterioration of stroke volume, low cardiac output, ECG abnormalities, decreased oxygen consumption and myocardial atrophy. Chronic heart disease may itself lead to malnutrition due to poor body tissue perfusion, hypoxia and hypermetabolism added to the lack of appetite caused by dyspnoea, hypomotility of the gastrointestinal tract, mental depression, distaste for sodium-restricted diets and lack of exercise.

The lung is also affected with atrophy of the respiratory muscles, deterioration in ventilatory mechanics, low vital capacity, depression of the hypoxic ventilatory response and respiratory failure.

Many patients with previous heart failure show cardiac cachexia, with no glycogen reserves in their tissues – especially the myocardium, the respiratory muscles and the liver. When they are subjected to cardiopulmonary bypass, they undergo massive metabolic changes, e.g. increased mobilization of endogenous substrates and carbohydrate stores, hydrolysis of triglycerides, lysis of protein for gluconeogenesis, and the effects of the hormones liberated during and after the operation.

Nutritional support may be offered by enteral and parenteral nutrition. The first is effective as long as the gastrointestinal tract is working normally. Unfortunately, in these patients with chronic malnutrition there is atrophy of intestinal villi and poor absorption. Furthermore, the concentration of some commercial compounds is high, the hyperosmolality causing diarrhoea. Parenteral nutrition, on the other hand, may overload the patient and is a possible source of infection due to the catheter and the solutions.

Neurological problems

Coma is the unwelcome evidence of neurological damage of diffuse type resulting from cardiac surgery; its depth and associated neurological signs suggest the likely outcome. Meanwhile, treatment is directed at the prevention of adverse consequences. The airway should be secure, lack of respiratory drive and cough reflexes and power should be compensated for artificially in the routine way (see later), and vasomotor instability watched for and treated according to the principles already mentioned, avoiding peripheral vasoconstriction and resultant cerebral consequences.

Nutrition should be via a nasogastric tube as soon as possible, with high nutrition intravenous feeding until then. Care of pressure areas, catheterization of the bladder, avoidance of corneal ulceration and suitable restraint to the restless patient are important.

Cultures should be taken regularly of sputum, urine, and any areas of broken skin including the wound, and antibiotics immediately given as appropriate.

Fits should be treated with phenytoin 200 mg stat and 50 mg 8-hourly intravenously with additional diazepam if necessary.

As soon as neurological damage is diagnosed, large doses of dexamethasone (10 mg i.v.) should be given, then 4 mg 6-hourly for three days to minimize the cerebral reaction. Oedema of the brain can also be reduced with diuretics – enough to mildly dehydrate the patient – and hyperosmolar colloidal infusions such as triple strength plasma or human albumin. Mannitol, sucrose or hypertonic saline may pass into the brain and then worsen oedema after initially improving it by taking water from the brain. Controlled hyperventilation and reduction of the body temperature in conjunction with a 'lytic cocktail' may improve the prospects for the brain cells.

Haematological problems

Postoperative bleeding is minimized by tidy surgery and ensuring a dry wound before closure, after as little bypass time as possible, in which as little transfused blood as possible has been used. Normal clotting reactions are shown in Figure 2.2.

Patients with deficient clotting factors, especially with polycythaemia, and those with a tendency to hypercoagulate and low cardiac output are more than normally prone to postoperative bleeding, while the likelihood of surgical bleeding is increased by connective tissue friability in such conditions as Marfan's syndrome.

Bleeding diseases like haemophilia, Christmas disease, abnormal platelets or abnormal capillaries should be diagnosed before surgery and treated. Surgery should be delayed for two weeks after aspirin if possible.

Platelet defects, defibrination, fibrinolysis, persistence of heparin, and shortage of factors V, VII, IX and X may develop during surgery. Full blood count, platelet count, prothrombin time (factors V, VII, X, II), kaolin-cephalin time (factors XII, XI, IX, VIII), bleeding time (platelets and capillary function), heparin protamine titration (residual heparin), fibrinogen level and Fi test (fibrinolysis) help to identify causes of postoperative bleeding.

While the tests are being done, replacement should be with fresh blood containing the factors V and VIII absent from older blood, which can get very depleted when large transfusions are given. If the haemoglobin is normal, fresh frozen plasma is a good first line of plasma volume replacement for the same reason.

If the tests show persistent heparin action, protamine should be given with further heparin titration control; intravascular coagulation producing defibrination is treated with heparin, and epsilon-aminocaproic acid (EACA) is the treatment for fibrinolysis, ensuring that heparin is given first if fibrinolysis co-exists with intravascular coagulation.

Low fibrinogen requires, of course, fibrinogen. Low prothrombin

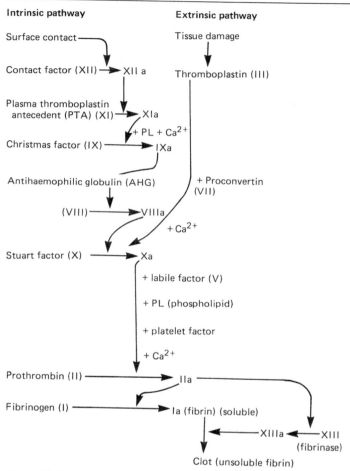

Figure 2.2 Coagulation cascade: clotting reactions. Notes: (1) a = 'active' form; (2) there is no Factor VI; (3) all the clotting factors except VIII (AHG) are formed in the liver

needs blood transfusion and vitamin K. Low platelets are supplemented with fresh blood or platelet transfusion.

Massive transfusion should be of fresh blood, warm and compensated for with $CaCl_2$ (3.5 ml of 10% solution for every unit of blood), re-opening when blood loss exceeds 300–400 ml/h or when there is a suspicion of cardiac tamponade.

Pyrexia

Though early central pyrexia is usually the result of lowered cardiac output with peripheral vasospasm and failure to lose central heat to the periphery, late pyrexia is suggestive of infection (in the wound, urine, chest or, worst of all, the bloodstream from a prosthesis).

All should be sent for culture; infected wounds should be opened and drained. All intravenous cannulae should be checked for phlebitis (strict asepsis should be observed in their management always) and any evoking redness removed. The deep veins of the leg should be checked for tenderness. If all these investigations are negative, drugs should be discontinued one by one if possible and blood cultures can then be repeated in the absence of antibiotics, as well as blood counts, film, Paul Bunnell, cytomegalovirus, hepatitis B antigen, antiheart antibodies, and other serology as indicated by local virology.

A diagnosis of 'post cardiotomy syndrome' is one of exclusion of infection and, when arrived at, indicates aspirin therapy or steroids if the first fails.

Liver failure

Peri-operative ischaemic hepatic damage is the likeliest cause of postoperative jaundice in those whose pre-operative hepatic function was normal, but other causes should be excluded.

Ischaemic damage of liver cells from low cardiac output produces a mixed obstructive and hepatocellular jaundice. There is also haemolysis of cells damaged by the heart-lung machine or the turbulence of paravalvular leaks, septal defects or malfunctioning prosthetic valves.

Jaundice is thus seen with multiorgan dysfunction – the sick cell syndrome. The real culprit is the malfunctioning heart and its inadequate output. However, the hepatic consequences must be treated. The liver needs adequate glucose and vitamins, and not too many fats, ethanol or hepatotoxic drugs or anaesthetic agents. Albumin may need to be supplemented intravenously, and coagulation must be checked, especially if the patient has to be on warfarin for a mechanical valve.

Neomycin may sterilize the gut and minimize portal venous bacteraemia, though the evidence for benefit was in dogs which normally have portal bacteraemia. Charcoal column haemodialysis or pig liver dialysis are desperate measures worthy of mention but probably not of action. Bowel washouts, oral protein restriction and neomycin may prevent the development of hepatic coma in toxic, pyrexial, profoundly generally ill, patients.

If total parental nutrition is necessary in liver failure, solutions without aromatic amino acids are mandatory, since aliphatic amino acids can be metabolized peripherally.

Late postoperative management

After discharge from the ITU, the return to twice daily check-overs by the house staff, twice weekly blood counts, electrolyte, prothrombin and enzyme assays, X-rays and electrocardiograms, should be gradual, the frequency of testing reducing as the situation stabilizes. Daily weighing should replace the scrupulous balance charts of the ITU as a means of assessing fluid balance and the need for diuretics. A portable ECG eases the transition from ITU monitoring to 6-hourly temperature and BP charts.

All mechanical valve replacements should have anticoagulation. As soon as the drains are removed, therefore, the loading dose of warfarin is given. Evidence suggests the long-term coronary graft patency rate is favourably influenced by soluble aspirin 75 mg twice weekly. An aspirin a day may help to prevent platelet thrombi forming on valves (which warfarin would not prevent), and aspirin/dipyridamole cover suffices for tissue valves.

Antibiotics are given prophylactically to open-heart patients over surgery. When no prosthesis is implanted, these are only necessary over the three days or so when drips and drains are still installed, whereas they should be given for two weeks with prostheses. Flucloxacillin provides cover against the more common (oral) bacteria. The short-term, narrow spectrum policy minimizes the risk of promoting multiresistant strains. Careful watch should be kept for fungal superinfection in sicker patients. Emphatic instruction should be given to all patients with prosthetic material implanted, to ensure that full antibiotic cover is given whenever any dental work is done or localized infections exist or urethral instrumentation performed.

Valve surgery

Varieties of prosthetic valves

Mechanical

- Starr Edwards (SE; Figure 2.3)
- Bjork Shiley (BSM; Figure 2.4)
- Lillehei-Kaster (LLK)
- Omniscience (OMI)
- Medtronic (MED)
- St Jude Medical (SJM)
- Duromedics (DM; Figure 2.5)

(1) *Silastic-balled valve* (the original design): mainly Starr Edwards which still is the basic standard. Better 'curing' of the silastic has prevented its deterioration.
(2) *Disc valve.* The discs are now made of pyrolite, which is almost diamond-hard carbon and has a negative surface charge. The differences are in the mode of retention of the disc, which can rotate and thus wears evenly. The different mounts permit various degrees of opening, 90° being the ideal as a well streamlined disc would be sideways on to the bloodstream and would provoke the least turbulence. Closure from this angle is unfortunately too slow and associated with an undue amount of regurgitation.

　　While silastic balls shed any clot that forms on them, disc

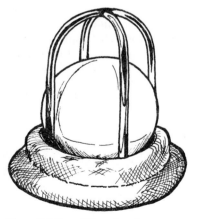

Figure 2.3 Starr Edwards valve

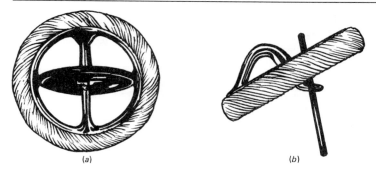

Figure 2.4 Bjork Shiley valve (*a*) from above; (*b*) lateral view

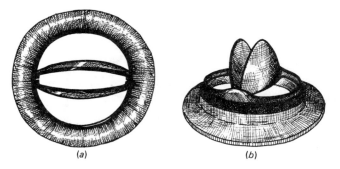

Figure 2.5 Duromedics valve (*a*) from above; (*b*) from below (no longer available)

valves would more likely accumulate the clot as a pannus which eventually traps the disc, so these valves are less obstructive to flow than ball valves, less likely to produce emboli but more likely to become 'frozen' by pannus. They include the Bjork Shiley, Lillehei-Kaster, and Hall Medtronics.

(3) *Double hemidisc valves*. These have the advantage of more laminar flow as the centrally hinged discs open fully and are side-on to the fastest part of the stream. They are all pyrolite (including the annulus) so are even less thrombogenic than pyrolite-disc-only valves. They have not been available as long as the other varieties so their long-term performance is not yet perfectly known. They are, however, the most promising hardware option. Examples are Duromedics, St Jude.

The most important disadvantage of mechanical valves is the need

for anticoagulation for their thrombogenicity. Also, their audibility
might make them poorly tolerated by the patient.

Biological

- Homograft
- Carpentier Edwards Porcine (CE; Figure 2.6*c* and *d*)
- Carpentier Edwards Pericardial (CEP)
- Carpentier Edwards Supra-annular (CES; Figure 2.6*a* and *b*)
- Ionescu Shiley (ISP)
- Mitral Medical Pericardial (MMP)
- Wessex Porcine (WP)
- Liotta (LI)
- Hancock (HA)
- Killingbeck (KLK)
- Tascon (TAS)

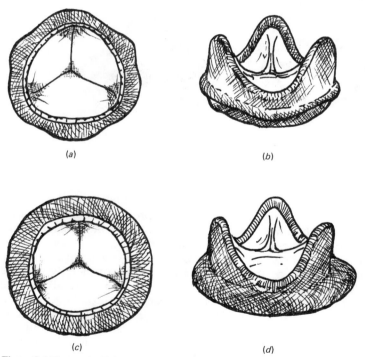

(a)

(b)

(c)

(d)

Figure 2.6 Carpentier Edwards supra-annular valve (*a*) from above; (*b*) from
below; (*c*) porcine valve from above; (*d*) from below

(1) *Human valves.* The original replacement for the aortic valve was human aortic valve. Nowadays, inserted after less than three weeks and kept in antibiotic medium, their performance is good, but skill and experience are necessary for insertion, which makes their use confined to centres where the necessary enthusiasm exists.

(2) *Porcine valves.* These are commercially available sewn to manu-factured mounting rings which make them affixable by the same techniques as all manufactured valves. They include Hancock, Liotta, Carpentier Edwards and Wessex. The variations are those of fixation and mount shape. All are fixed at low tension which keeps the collagen more 'crinkly' and flexible.

(3) *Pericardial valves.* This pattern is biological in that it is glutar-aldehyde-fixed pericardium but handcrafted into cusp form with some resultant benefit to haemodynamic performance. The Ionescu Shiley, Mitral Medical Pericardial and Carpentier Edwards Pericardial are the main brands of this type.

All these biological valves are minimally thrombogenic and can thus be used without anticoagulants in those patients wishing to have pregnancies or to boldly go where no anticoagulant is available. Their durability is the unknown fact – so far it appears that they will last between five and ten years.

Mitral stenosis

This is always related to rheumatic fever and presents with dysp-noea, pulmonary oedema, arrhythmias or embolism.

Medical treatment is based on diuretics, sodium restriction, digoxin, beta blockers and treatment of complications (arrhythmias, peripheral embolism, haemoptysis, infection).

Surgery is indicated if the stenosis is severe, in the presence of pulmonary hypertension (critical area: less than $1.5\,cm^2$) or if there is heavy calcification or extreme symptoms. Commissurotomy is indi-cated in non-calcified pure mitral stenosis. Otherwise mitral valve replacement is performed with a mechanical valve unless the patient is old, if pregnancy is expected or if anticoagulation is contra-indicated, when a bioprosthetic valve is inserted.

Mitral incompetence

This is the most common valve lesion and may be primary (rheuma-tic fever, bacterial endocarditis, chordal or papillary muscle damage or cusp redundancy) or secondary to aortic valve disease or cardio-myopathy.

Once the cause has been controlled, treatment with vasodilators (hydralazine, captopril, prazosin) in order to reduce the afterload, as well as diuretics, digoxin and inotropics if the patient is in heart failure, may suffice. Prophylaxis for infective endocarditis is important, particularly when dental procedures, active infections or surgery are anticipated.

Surgery is indicated in refractory heart failure and when other surgical heart diseases are present (coronary artery disease).

Aortic stenosis

Aortic stenosis may be congenital, degenerative or inflammatory. Its symptoms may start late in the course of the disease, but after the first episode of angina, syncope, dyspnoea or heart failure, death will come in 50% within two years.

The treatment is mechanical correction. It is conservative (surgical or percutaneous valvuloplasty) in congenital aortic stenosis or in non-calcified disease. Otherwise aortic valve replacement is mandatory. A gradient greater than 30 mmHg and a valve orifice smaller than 1 cm² indicate significant stenosis.

If the annulus is small a double disc valve is recommended, unless the patient is a female in active sexual life or if anticoagulation is contraindicated, in which case a bioprosthetic valve is the choice.

Aortic incompetence

The main problem here is left ventricular volume overload with congestive heart failure.

Medical treatment should be started provided there is not progressively increasing heart size, pulmonary embolism or severe ventricular dilatation on echocardiography.

Emergency surgery is indicated in acute incompetence due to infective endocarditis, particularly if vegetations or aortic root abscess are present. Also, if pulmonary oedema, septal involvement by the infection (heart block), renal failure or fungal endocarditis are diagnosed.

Tricuspid valve disease

This is generally secondary to mitral or aortic valve disease. Nevertheless, it can be affected by intravenously introduced endocarditis, rheumatic fever and carcinoid syndrome. When advanced or organic, severe right heart failure is present.

It is best assessed during operation as it is very rare for the triscuspid valve to fail primarily. According to the severity of the disease, a valvuloplasty (Carpentier ring or De Vega annuloplasty) is indicated, but in severe primary disease the valve should be replaced.

Problems associated with valve surgery

In *closed mitral valvotomy* the main problem is thromboembolism. If the valve is calcified or a big clot is found in the atrium, the procedure should be abandoned for an open valvotomy. Other possible problems are:

● bleeding from ventricular or atrial incisions
● severe regurgitation from excessive tension and tearing of cusp
● incomplete valvotomy (suggested by low cardiac output and pulmonary oedema in the postoperative period).

Open mitral valve repair could be complicated by:
● valve damage (dilated ring, cusp damage or ruptured chordae)
● air embolism
● thromboembolism.

Mitral valve replacement can cause severe problems when the prosthesis is attached to an incompletely prepared valve ring or one too attenuated by excessive calcium removal. Other possible problems include:
● imperfect resection of the subvalvular apparatus (too little: valvular jam; too much: ventricular perforation)
● paravalvular leak
● disruption of the atrioventricular junction (generally lethal and resulting from over-excision of the mitral valve ring, deep sutures, too large prosthesis or excessive surgical lifting)
● damage to the aortic valve
● heart block
● damage to the circumflex coronary artery by over-deep sutures.

Aortic valve replacement may cause:
● calcium embolism
● heart block
● paravalvular leak
● bleeding from the aorta
● heart failure due to intra-operative cardiac damage
● valve malfunction.

Tricuspid valve replacement may be complicated by heart block due to the proximity of its septal leaflet to the bundle of His. Also, thrombosis and refractory right heart failure.

Some complications related to valve surgery are:

(1) Post-perfusion syndrome (2–8 weeks after surgery, presenting with fever, splenomegaly, lymphocytosis and neutropenia).
(2) Post-pericardiotomy syndrome (polyserositis four weeks after the operation presenting with temperature, pleuritis, myalgias, leukocytosis and pericarditis).
(3) Blood trauma (mainly by mechanical valves in the aortic position) with haemolysis and anaemia.
(4) Thrombosis, mostly associated with mechanical valves, may cause severe valve malfunction and systemic or pulmonary embolism.
(5) Prosthetic endocarditis, in the form of vegetations or abscesses presenting as sepsis, embolism and heart failure.
(6) Valve dysfunction or perivalvular or valvular leak leading to valve failure.

Later complications are:
● calcification
● late thrombosis
● degeneration
● tearing of cusps
● adverse effects of anticoagulants and antiplatelet therapy.

Infective endocarditis

In this intravascular and disseminated form of infection the most common microorganisms isolated are: *Streptococcus viridans* (40–50%); *Streptococcus* B (10–20%); *Staphylococcus aureus* (10–15%); *Staphylococcus epidermidis* (5–10%); Gram negative bacilli (6–8%); negative culture (8–12%). In cases of prosthetic valve infective endocarditis the frequency changes to streptococci, *Staphylococcus aureus*, Gram-negative bacilli and uncommon microorganisms like *Candida*.

The immune system is affected with the presence of circulating immune complexes, low complement levels and hyperimmuno-globulinaemia.

There are two clinical phases – one of acute endocarditis with embolic manifestations and low level of circulating immune complexes and a chronic one of high levels of circulating immune complexes. The most important prognostic factors are:

(a) mode of onset;
(b) duration of illness;
(c) infecting microorganisms;
(d) renal complications;
(e) CNS complications;
(f) haemodynamic deterioration;
(g) positivity of cultures after treatment.

It may present with heart failure, sepsis or peripheral embolism, plus signs of aortic or mitral incompetence in the presence of cutaneous signs, glomerulonephritis and/or mycotic aneurysms. In cases of triscuspid involvement (in drug addicts or immunocompromised patients), the septic signs along with lung infiltrates suggest the diagnosis.

Treatment includes specific antibiotics, medications for heart failure, treatment of complications and surgery.

Operation is indicated by haemodynamic deterioration, valve failure, persistent sepsis, systemic embolism and uncommon microorganisms.

Prosthetic endocarditis, usually after dental or surgical procedures without antibiotic coverage, presents with signs of prosthetic valve leakage demonstrated by echocardiography.

Heart muscle diseases

Cardiomyopathies

(1) *Dilated (95%)*. Characterized by weak systole, slow diastole, thin wall and big cavity. The cause is unknown in most cases. Specific causes are:

- valvular disease
- pericardial disease
- coronary artery disease
- myocarditis
- vitamin deficiencies
- thyroid disease
- alcoholism
- drugs
- sarcoidosis
- parturition.

Clinically dilated cardiomyopathies may have tricuspid incompetence and mitral incompetence with huge residual volumes and small ejection fractions. These do worst. Those with more muscular hypertrophy do better. Cardiac biopsy may help to diagnose any specific muscle disease. The therapeutic options are:

- bed rest
- diuretics
- potassium supplements
- digoxin
- vasodilators
- anti-arrhythmic agents
- immunosuppressors (azathioprine, prednisone, cyclosporin)
- cardiac transplant.

(2) *Hypertrophic.* Presents with strong systole, slow diastole, thick wall and small cavity. Treatment is based on correcting any specific cause like hypertension, subaortic stenosis, aortic stenosis, coarctation of the aorta, etc. The cause is unknown in most cases and the treatment is based on disopyramide, calcium antagonists, beta blockers and, in some cases, ventriculomyectomy.

(3) *Restrictive.* Presents with normal systole, slow and limited diastole, normal wall and normal cavity. Its causes are:

- endomyocardial fibrosis
- carcinoid syndrome
- drugs, e.g. methysergide
- glycogen diseases
- amyloidosis
- haemochromatosis
- Chagas' disease.

Endomyocardial fibrosis is recognized when left and right ventricles show apical obliteration or well contracting ventricles with high filling pressures. Atrioventricular valve incompetence is common and eosinophilia may be present.

The investigations recommended may be aetiological and functional. Exclude haemochromatosis, collagen disease, immunological disease, acromegaly, porphyria, phaeochromocytoma, beri-beri, alcoholism, specific infections, peripheral muscle disease, and amyloidosis. Haemodynamic investigations should be carried out to exclude pericardial effusion or constriction, myxoma, left or right atrial obliteration or pulmonary hypertension, coronary artery disease. Right heart catheter with pulmonary arteriogram exposed to show left side of the heart as well. Left sided pictures free from ectopics in order to show the size of the left ventricular cavity in systole and in diastole and the thickness of the left ventricular wall.

Acute myopericarditis

In acute situations it should be assumed that there is a combination of muscle and pericardium inflammation in primary muscle disease. But pericarditis causes secondary inflammation of the myocardium, so the term myopericarditis is now preferred.

The aetiology includes:

- transplant rejection
- virus (ECHO, polio, coxsackie)
- bacteria (cocci, *Clostridium, Brucella*)
- *Mycoplasma*
- parasitic (trichinosis)
- protozoal (*Trypanosoma, Toxoplasma*)
- rickettsial
- fungal.

Drug-induced myopericarditis is classified in two groups:

(1) Primary myocardium forms: sulphonamides, tetracyclines, methyldopa, cytostatic agents, lithium, emetine and antimony.
(2) Primary pericardial forms: procainamide; hydralazine, isoniazid, penicillin, methysergide, streptomycin and phenylbutazone amongst others.

Biopsy may help in unexplained heart failure, unexplained ventricular arrhythmias, suspected myocarditis and to monitor or to exclude rejection.

Cardiac transplantation

The main indication for cardiac transplantation is terminal heart disease with failure refractory to medical and surgical treatment and with a life expectancy of less than one year without transplant. Causes include:

(a) cardiomyopathies;
(b) ischaemic heart disease;
(c) valvular heart disease;
(d) myocarditis;

(e)   non-malignant cardiac tumours;
(f)   some congenital malformations;
(g)   massive coronary embolism;
(h)   sequelae of trauma.

The most important contraindications for the procedure are:

(a)   pulmonary vascular hypertension (more than 6 units Wood or more than 600 dyne/cm^{-5});
(b)   insulin-dependent diabetes mellitus;
(c)   active infection;
(d)   hepatic failure;
(e)   renal failure;
(f)   recent pulmonary embolism;
(g)   collagen disease;
(h)   cardiac cachexia;
(i)   age over 55 years;
(j)   psychosocial instability.

The donor should be below the age of 35 years and there should be no previous heart disease, cardiac trauma, extensive cardiac massage, prolonged hypotension, abnormal ECG, low cardiac output, active infection or massive doses of inotropics to maintain the cardiac output. The ischaemic period (counted from the aortic cross clamping) must be less than 4 h with adequate cardioplegia. The donor should also have a similar corporeal mass to the recipient.

Histocompatibility is assessed by testing the recipient blood, which should be the same group as the donor. Also, the recipient's serum must be tested against donor lymphocytes seeking cytotoxic antibodies. Anaesthetic management includes strict aseptic technique, pre-operative antibiotics (flucloxacillin 2 g or lincomycin 1.2 g) and, in some centres, antithymocytic globulin (10 mg/kg diluted in 125 ml of normal saline at 30 ml/h). Every blood product must be CMV negative.

Postoperative management

Before removing the aortic clamp the inotropics are started (isoprenaline: 3 µg/kg/min; dopamine: 3 µg/kg/min; sodium nitroprusside: 10 µg/kg/min; and adrenaline if required).

Once the patient is off bypass, methylprednisolone (500 mg i.v.), frusemide (20 mg i.v.), flucloxacillin (1 g), calcium chloride (10 mmol) and mannitol 25% (25 ml in 25 min) are administered.

Postoperative management should include barrier nursing, early extubation, early removal of catheters and lines, and early mobilization.

Pre-operative cyclosporin is given in a dose of 4–8 mg/kg, depending on the creatinine clearance. Postoperatively it is measured by radioimmunoassay, keeping serum levels between 100–300 ng/ml for the first month, and 50–150 ng/ml afterwards.

Other postoperative drugs are:

- Azathioprine: 4 mg/kg start dose and then 1–3 mg/kg/day to keep the white count between 4000 and 6000/mm^3.
- Antithymocytic immunoglobulin: 10 mg/day for 7 days.
- Steroids: methylprednisolone, 500 mg at the end of bypass and then 125 mg i.v. 12-hourly for 36 h. Prednisolone is started 12 h after the last doses of methylprednisolone, at 0.5 mg/kg starting dose and then from 0.8 mg/kg on the third day to 0.2 mg/kg on the seventh day and afterwards.

Rejection is detected by routine endomyocardial biopsy and is treated by methylprednisolone (pulse therapy: 1 g i.v. daily for 3 days). If severe rejection is found on biopsy, antithymocytic globulin at 7 mg/kg infusion for 14 days is given.

If infection is suspected, an urgent biopsy is performed and tests for common bacteria, virus (CMV and herpes), fungi (*Coccidioides, Cryptococcus*) and *Toxoplasma* are done.

Other complications are:

- accelerated atherosclerosis
- malignant diseases from immunosuppression
- hypertension
- renal failure
- hepatic failure
- convulsions
- interstitial myocardial fibrosis.

Aortic aneurysms

Ascending aortic aneurysm

The patient may present in heart failure with signs of aortic incompetence. If found incidentally on echocardiography, less than 6 cm and without aortic regurgitation, observation and medical treatment is indicated. If bigger than 6 cm or if aortic incompetence is found, surgery is advisable. If the aortic valve is normal, a tube graft is inserted..Otherwise aortic valve replacement with aneurysm-orrhaphy, supracoronary tube graft or valve conduit with coronary re-implantation are choices.

Descending thoracic aortic aneurysm

Aneurysms greater than 6 cm on CT scan or aortogram should be replaced. If the aneurysm is localized and renal and mesenteric function are normal, a temporary bypass from the ascending aorta to the descending aorta, or from left atrium to left femoral artery before the aortic replacement, may diminish the risk of spinal injury if the femoral pressure falls below 30 mmHg when the aorta is cross clamped.

Other indications for surgery in aortic aneurysms are:

- proximal dissection involving the coronary arteries
- cardiac tamponade
- progressive organ failure
- impending rupture
- severe and intractable pain
- severe hypotension.

Additional measures include pain relief and control of hypertension (see Hypertensive emergencies, p. 27).

Aortic dissection

Dissection of the ascending aorta

Once myocardial infarction is ruled out, chest X-rays and CT scan will show enlargement of the ascending aorta. Angiography will delimit the length of dissection but CT scan is more sensitive to diagnosis. If the patient's condition is too poor or if the brain has been badly affected, medical therapy is continued. Otherwise, operation may be:

(1) Aortic valve replacement and graft replacement of the ascending aorta.
(2) Tube graft to the ascending aorta.
(3) 'Sandwich' oversewing of the origin of the dissection.

Dissection of the descending aorta

CT scan, chest X-rays and angiography (contrast or digital substraction) will show the extent of the disease.

If the patient is *in extremis*, medical therapy is continued. If fit for operation and there is a short length of dissection, clamping and suture is indicated. Otherwise left atrium-left femoral bypass, or aortofemoral Gott shunt is indicated before any procedure.

Antihypertensives and beta blockers may have replaced emergency surgery for dissection of the aorta in patients whose prospects of surviving six weeks, when 'cold' surgery can be done, are greater with drugs than surgery. An escalating regime of antihypertensive agents (see Hypertensive emergencies, p. 27), together with analgesia and sedation as well as diuretics and strict monitoring may delay the need for surgery until the condition improves. The first choice of drugs is beta blockers which reduce dp/dt and systolic pressure, rather than vasodilators which may increase pulse pressure by lowering diastolic pressure. Only when full beta blockade is accomplished should next-line therapy be relied upon, which should be acetylcholinesterase inhibition and sodium deprivation.

Surgery should be done when complications of the dissection (vital arteries occluding or aortic valve regurgitation) threaten survival.

Congenital Heart Disease

Cardiac arrest in children

(1) Clear airway.
(2) Ventilation: mouth to mouth; bag to mouth; intubation (Figure 3.1)
    Tube size: Small neonates: 3 mm
                Large neonates: 3.5 mm
                6 months: 4 mm
                1 year: 4.5 mm
                3 years: 5 mm
                5 years: 5.5 mm
                7 years: 6 mm
                10 years: 6.5 mm
                15 years: 7 mm.
(3) Cardiac massage. If not effective, rule out oesophageal intubation, severe hypovolaemia, tracheal obstruction, pneumothorax, cardiac tamponade.
(4) Sodium bicarbonate (8.4% = 1 mmol per 1 ml): 1 ml/kg start dose and further doses of 0.5 ml/kg every 10 min of arrest.
(5) Define asystole, fibrillation, electromechanical dissociation.
(6) Adrenaline (1:10000 solution): 0.1–0.2 ml/kg or 10–20 µg/kg.
    Small neonate: 0.25 ml
    Large neonate: 0.5 ml
    6 months: 0.75 ml
    1 year: 1 ml
    3 years: 1.5 ml
    5 years: 2 ml
    7 years: 2.5 ml
    10 years: 3 ml
    15 years: 5 ml.
(7) Defibrillation: 2–4 J/kg.
(8) Check cardiac output. Use drugs according to:
    Preload. Too low: volume; too high: diuretics, vasodilators.
    Afterload. Too low: adrenaline; too high: vasodilators.

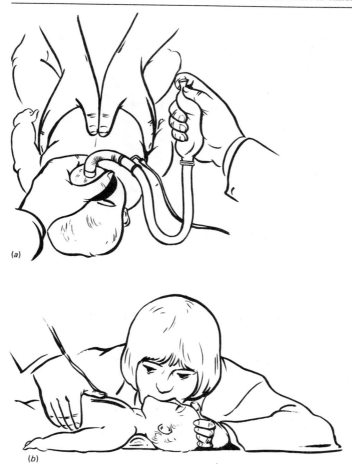

Figure 3.1 (*a*) and (*b*) Cardiac resuscitation in children

      Myocardium: sympathomimetics.
(9) Other drugs:
      Atropine: 0.1–0.6 mg i.v.
      Calcium gluconate: 10–20 mg/kg
      Frusemide: 1 mg/kg
      Lignocaine: 1 mg/kg
(10) Reduce cerebral oedema: frusemide, mannitol, hyperventilation.
(11) Reduce cerebral oxygen requirements: cooling, barbiturates.

(12) Infusions:

      Adrenaline (0.15–0.3 µg/kg/min)
        5 mg/500 ml = 10 µg/ml = 1–2 ml/kg/h
      Noradrenaline (0.10–0.15 µg/kg/min)
        3 mg/500 ml = 6 µg/ml = 1–1.5 ml/kg/h
      Isoprenaline (0.1–0.5 µg/kg/min
        2 mg/500 ml = 4 µg/ml = 0.3–1.5 ml/kg/h
      Dopamine (5–20 µg/kg/min)
        200 mg/500 ml = 400 µg/ml = 0.75–3 ml/kg/h
      Dobutamine (2.5–10 µg/kg/min)
        250 mg/500 ml = 500 µg/ml = 0.3–1.2 ml/kg/h
      Salbutamol (0.1–0.5 µg/kg/min)
        5 mg/500 ml = 10 µg/ml = 0.5–3.0 ml/kg/h

The child with congenital heart disease

The initial symptoms are usually failure to thrive, dyspnoea, respiratory infections, cardiac murmur and cyanosis.

Chest X-rays show cardiomegaly and lung congestion, ECG shows chamber enlargement and echocardiography gives detailed information on the particular anatomy of the malformation, which is confirmed by angiography.

Patients may be divided into two groups, cyanotic and acyanotic, and each group subdivided according to the amount of pulmonary blood flow.

Acyanotic

Normal or moderately increased pulmonary blood flow (vessel marking)

(1) With left ventricular enlargement:
- Ventricular septal defect (VSD)
- Atrial septal defect (ASD)
- Patent ductus arteriosus (PDA)

(2) With right ventricular enlargement:
- Atrial septal defect (ASD)
- Partial anomalous pulmonary venous drainage (PAPVD)

Increased pulmonary blood flow

(1) With left ventricular enlargement:
- Aortic stenosis (AS)
- Mitral regurgitation (MR)
- Coarctation of the aorta (CoAo)

(2) With right ventricular enlargement:
- Mitral stenosis (MS)

Cyanotic

Increased pulmonary blood flow

(1) With left ventricular enlargement:
- Truncus arteriosus (TA)
- Single ventricle (SV)
- Transposition of the great arteries (TGA)
(2) With right ventricular enlargement:
- Total anomalous pulmonary venous drainage (TAPVD)
- Transposition of great arteries (TGA)
- Hypoplastic left ventricle (Hyp LV)

Decreased pulmonary blood flow

(1) With left ventricular enlargement:
- Truncus arteriosus (TA)
- Hypoplastic right ventricle (Hyp RV)
(2) With biventricular enlargement:
- Transposition of the great arteries with pulmonary stenosis
(3) With right ventricular enlargement:
- Ebstein malformation (EM)
- Tetralogy of Fallot (TOF)

Congenital heart defects

Patent ductus arteriosus (PDA)

The ductus usually closes physiologically 12 h after birth. It is usually asymptomatic, but in premature babies may present with congestive heart failure. The most important clinical finding is the continuous murmur.

Initial treatment of patients in heart failure due to PDA is with indomethacin (0.2 mg/kg) through a nasogastric tube in order to block prostaglandin synthetase and to promote PDA closure.

Surgery is contraindicated when there is Eisenmenger syndrome (reversal of flow due to severe pulmonary hypertension). Surgical procedure is ligation or division of PDA.

Other contraindications for PDA closure are pulmonary atresia, pulmonary stenosis and coarctation of the aorta, unless surgery includes correction of all the anomalies.

Complications include infection, pulmonary haemorrhage and ligation of the pulmonary artery.

Atrial septal defect (ASD)

ASD is generally asymptomatic or presents with recurrent chest infections. On examination, an ejection systolic murmur over the pulmonary area and fixed splitting of the second sound may be noticed. It also may present with pulmonary hypertension, heart failure and arrhythmias.

ASD can be:

(1) Secundum type: in the mid-portion of the septum
(2) Primum type: associated with mitral and tricuspid valve defects
(3) Sinus venosus: high in the septum and associated with partial anomalous pulmonary venous drainage
(4) Coronary sinus

The most common type is the secundum type and surgery is indicated if significant shunt (Qp/Qs ratio > 1.5/1.0). Some centres operate on ASD routinely because of the possibility of further complications, e.g. arrhythmias, paradoxical embolism, etc.

The primum type is a more serious disease because of its association with anomalies of the atrioventricular valves, as part of the spectrum of atrioventricular septal defect.

In the sinus venosus type the right superior pulmonary vein is connected with the superior vena cava. Every case should be assessed individually to decide if direct suture or patch with repair of associated anomalies is necessary.

Surgical complications are heart block, arrhythmias, endocarditis and repair failure.

Atrioventricular canal defects

An abnormal development of atrial and ventricular septum involving tricuspid and mitral valves. It is partial if there is ASD with cleft anterior mitral leaflet, complete if there is VSD, ASD, cleft mitral valve and cleft tricuspid valve.

Treatment is surgical and usually through the right atrium. The common mitral and tricuspid leaflets are separated, the mitral valve is repaired, the ASD and VSD closed with a common patch and the valve leaflets attached to it.

Coarctation of the aorta

This condition may be asymptomatic or show a picture of heart failure, respiratory distress and failure to thrive. There is also hypertension of the upper part of the body with specific X-ray signs (notched ribs). Angiography is necessary if associated malformations are suspected and balloon dilatation can be attempted.

Initial treatment is directed to control hypertension and heart failure. Types of repair are:

- subclavian patch aortoplasty (Walhausen)
- resection and end-to-end anastomosis
- patch arterioplasty
- prosthetic replacement
- bypass with the subclavian artery or with graft.

Postoperative complications are paraplegia, paradoxical hypertension and re-coarctation.

Ventricular septal defect (VSD)

This is one of the commonest cardiac malformations. If there is a big shunt (more than 1.5:1) and/or elevated pulmonary resistance, surgery is indicated. There are five types of VSD:

(1) Subaortic (in the outlet septum).
(2) Supracristal (underneath the pulmonary artery).
(3) Infracristal:
    (a) AV canal type;
    (b) muscular;
    (c) apical.

The left ventricle and the right atrium may also communicate (Gerbode).

In relation to the aortic root diameter, the VSD may be small (less than 40%), moderate (40–60%) and large. The defect can be closed transatrially, transventricularly (if muscle bridges are to be resected), through the pulmonary artery (supracristal defects) and transaortically (subaortic defects).

If the patient is too small, or in severe heart failure, or if multiple defects are present, pulmonary artery banding may be attempted before closure.

Aortopulmonary septal defect

These babies present with early heart failure and a machinery murmur. There are three different types of defect:

(1) Aorta–main pulmonary artery above the sinus of Valsalva.
(2) Aorta–terminal portion of main pulmonary artery.
(3) Aorta–right pulmonary artery.

Surgical treatment is patching under cardiopulmonary bypass in type 1, patching under total cardiocirculatory arrest in type 2, and complete detachment of the right pulmonary artery in type 3.

Total anomalous pulmonary venous drainage

These patients are treated initially with ventilation, correction of acidosis, nutrition, prostaglandin E_1 (in order to keep the ductus open) and transatrial septostomy (Rashkind procedure).

Operation is performed according to the type of defect:

(1) Cardiac type under cardiopulmonary bypass: the blood is diverted from the pulmonary veins to the left atrium by sectioning the coronary sinus wall.
(2) Supracardiac and infracardiac: both types are treated by anastomosing the common pulmonary vein to the left atrium.

The ASD and the PDA are also closed.

Tetralogy of Fallot

This consists of a VSD, right ventricular outflow tract obstruction, right ventricular hypertrophy and overriding of the aorta over the ventricles. The critical problem is the degree of pulmonary stenosis and the diminished pulmonary blood flow. The patient is usually cyanotic, with various degrees of heart failure, dyspnoea, squatting and hypoxic spells.

The spectrum varies from mild pulmonary stenosis to complete pulmonary atresia and the main types are:

(1) Pulmonary arteries of good size, infundibular stenosis and pulmonary valvular stenosis.
(2) Narrow pulmonary artery with good sized branches.
(3) Small and narrow pulmonary artery and branches.
(4) Pulmonary atresia.

Indications for operation are cyanotic spells, haematocrit higher than 60%, resting oxygen saturation less than 70%, refractory heart failure.

Initially, prostaglandin E_1 (PGE_1) is given to maintain the ductus open. When surgery is decided, the options available, in addition to closure of the VSD are:

(a) simple pulmonary valvotomy;
(b) right ventricular outflow patch;
(c) right ventricle to pulmonary artery conduit.

If open operation has to be delayed for any reason, a temporary aortopulmonary shunt (Blalock Taussig or Waterston) or a closed pulmonary valvotomy is performed.

Truncus arteriosus

The aorta and the pulmonary artery originate in a common trunk. A large VSD is usually present. There are four types:

Type I. Pulmonary artery trunk coming from the aorta.
Type II. The two branches of the pulmonary artery originate from the aorta separately but not widely apart one from the other.
Type III. The two branches of the pulmonary artery originate, widely separated, from the aorta.
Type IV. No pulmonary artery branches or small ones arising from the distal aorta.

If symptoms are moderate and there is no pulmonary hypertension, operation may be delayed. If there is heart failure resistant to medical treatment, including aggressive vasodilatation, pulmonary artery banding may delay open surgery until the child is larger. Operation may consist of VSD closure redirecting the left ventricular flow to the aorta, separation of the pulmonary trunk, closure of the right ventricular outflow tract and anastomosis of this trunk to the right ventricle through an external conduit (Rastelli procedure).

Pulmonary atresia with VSD

May be considered part of the spectrum of tetralogy of Fallot. There are five main types:

(1) Infundibular muscle obstruction.
(2) Imperforate valve.
(3) Short atretic segment.
(4) Long atretic segment.
(5) Complete atresia.

If the patient is cyanotic, PGE_1 is given to maintain the ductus open before a pulmonary-systemic shunt is performed.

Pulmonary atresia with intact ventricular septum

There is hypoplasia of the right ventricle. The patient is cyanotic from birth.

After PGE_1 is administered to keep the ductus open, balloon atrial septostomy is performed at the time of catheterization (Rashkind procedure). Afterwards, a systemic to pulmonary shunt is indicated. In cases of extremely hypoplastic right ventricle, atrial septectomy (Blalock Hanlon procedure), systemic-pulmonary shunt and pulmonary valvotomy are the best choices.

Once the presence of right ventricular infundibulum is established, pulmonary valvotomy (Brock type) or right ventricular outflow patch are attempted. Otherwise a Fontan procedure (anastomosis right atrium-pulmonary artery) should be carried out.

Ebstein anomaly

This is the combination of low tricuspid valve attachment with right ventricular hypoplasia, tricuspid incompetence and ASD.

Tricuspid valve repair or replacement with ASD closure may control the problem. An alternative is a Glenn-Patiño shunt (termino-lateral anastomosis of the SVC to the right pulmonary artery) if the right ventricle is obstructed. Afterwards, a Fontan procedure is performed.

Congenital aortic stenosis

The critical gradient is 50 mmHg. Valvotomy or valvuloplasty is indicated if this gradient is greater than 70 mmHg or if the orifice area is less than 0.4 cm^2/m^2 body surface area.

If supravalvular stenosis is present, a patch aortoplasty is required. In valvular stenosis, aortic valvotomy or percutaneous valvuloplasty is the choice. In subvalvular stenosis, resection of the fibromuscular membrane will relieve the obstruction.

Other alternatives in specific cases are: aortic valve replacement; Konno procedure (aortoplasty enlarging the aortic annulus and the ventricular septum with patch closure and aortic valve replacement); left ventricle to aorta conduit.

Hypoplastic left heart

There is atresia of aortic and mitral valves and hypoplasia of the left ventricle. The patient is characteristically pale and in severe heart failure.

Initial medical treatment is followed by palliative procedures, e.g. Norwood operation (creation of a truncus arteriosus and atrial septectomy), Fontan procedure.

Univentricular heart

If no outlet chamber is present or if the outlet chamber is below the pulmonary artery with excessive pulmonary artery flow, pulmonary banding is performed. If the outlet chamber is below the pulmonary artery and the flow is restricted, a Blalock Taussig shunt is done before a Fontan procedure.

If there is associated transposition of the great arteries, there are various choices:

(a) septation (if good pulmonary flow);
(b) Blalock shunt (if restricted pulmonary flow);
(c) Norwood (if subaortic stenosis).

The Fontan procedure is the definitive one.

Cor triatriatum

The left atrium is divided into two by a fibrous membrane. An ASD is present above or below this membrane. The patient presents with heart failure.

Treatment is excision of the membrane and ASD closure.

Aneurysm of the sinus of Valsalva

This may be associated with fistula from the aorta to the right atrium or right ventricle. It is clinically asymptomatic unless a fistula is present, in which case chest pain, dyspnoea, heart failure and a continuous murmur are present.

If there is no rupture the aneurysm is repaired from the aorta by patch closure. If a fistula is present the defect is closed from the ventricle, which is more convenient when VSD is also present, or with rather more security through the aorta and the ventricle simultaneously.

Double outlet right ventricle

Both great arteries originate from the ventricle (usually one complete artery and 50% of the other). According to the location of the associated VSD, this syndrome may be divided into:

(a) subaortic
(b) non-committed
(c) subpulmonary (Taussig Bing if the aorta is to the right).

The subaortic type can be corrected by a Kirklin procedure

(intraventricular tunnel from the VSD to the aorta, redirecting the flow). The non-committed VSD is more difficult to repair and might be inoperable. The subpulmonary VSD with aorta and pulmonary artery side by side is approached by a Yacoub procedure (resection of the infundibular septum and tunnel from the VSD to the aorta posteriorly to the pulmonary outflow tract). Another alternative is the Abe procedure (tubular prosthesis from VSD to aorta).

If the aorta is anterior to the subpulmonary VSD, it is connected to the pulmonary artery creating in that way a transposition, with subsequent Senning, Mustard or Jatene operations.

Interrupted aortic arch

There is segmental atresia of the aortic arch, associated with PDA and VSD. It can be distal to the left subclavian artery, between the left common carotid and the left subclavian, and between the innominate and left common carotid arteries.

Treatment is surgical by resection and anastomosis, conduit or bypass using the subclavian artery. Associated procedures include VSD closure, PDA ligation and/or pulmonary banding.

Transposition of the great arteries

The aorta originates from the right ventricle and the pulmonary artery from the left ventricle, with two separated circulations joined by an additional defect (ASD, VSD, PDA), without which the patient would not survive.

Initial treatment is a Rashkind procedure (balloon atrial septostomy) and PGE_1 is administered to keep the ductus opened. Later, atrial septectomy (Blalock Hanlon) may be another preliminary step before correction. If there is a VSD with increased pulmonary flow, pulmonary artery banding is carried out. If there is a VSD with pulmonary stenosis, an aorto-pulmonary shunt (Blalock Taussig) is performed, followed by a Rastelli procedure (patch closure of the VSD with flow redirection from left ventricle to aorta and conduit from right ventricle to pulmonary artery).

Definitive correction is by intra-atrial rearrangement of the blood flow (Senning, Mustard) or by arterial switch (with coronary switch: Jatene; without coronary switch: Damus-Stansel-Kaye procedure).

Vascular rings

This refers to aortic arch malformations compromising the upper respiratory tract and the oesophagus, causing respiratory distress, recurrent respiratory infections and dysphagia.

The first diagnostic step is an oesophagogram. Then angiography will confirm the abnormal anatomy. Through a left thoracotomy the branches are identified. If the cause is a ligamentum arteriosum, it is divided. If a double aortic arch is present, the smaller one is divided. If an aberrant right subclavian artery, it is also divided.

Systemic-pulmonary shunts

These are performed to improve pulmonary blood flow, tissue oxygenation and pulmonary artery growth.

Types:

(1) Blalock Taussig: subclavian artery to pulmonary artery.
(2) Waterston: right pulmonary artery to ascending aorta.
(3) Cooley-Potts-Smith: left pulmonary artery to descending aorta.
(4) Glenn-Patiño: superior vena cava to right pulmonary artery.

Respiratory Medicine

Admission procedure in thoracic non-cardiac cases

The main symptoms of respiratory disease are:

(1) Cough – if persistent, painful and productive.
(2) Sputum production.
(3) Haemoptysis.
(4) Breathlessness – implies loss of pulmonary function.
(5) Wheeze – airways obstruction.
(6) Chest pain – implies pleural involvement.

Signs to look for are:

(1) Finger clubbing.
(2) Central cyanosis.
(3) Stridor.
(4) Chest movements, expansion and shape.
(5) Abnormal percussion (dullness, solid lungs or pleural fluid).
(6) Auscultation:
   ● bronchial breathing (consolidation);
   ● aegophony (level of pleural effusion);
   ● rhonchi, rales (airway narrowing, sputum);
   ● crepitations (oedema).

The chest X-ray may reveal abnormalities of ribs, pleurae, diaphragm and mediastinum which should be sought before looking at the lung parenchyma. Both projections, anteroposterior and lateral, should be examined. Also lung function tests, special diagnostic procedures and CT scan may be indicated.

Respiratory function tests

Ventilatory mechanics

(1) Maximum voluntary ventilation.
(2) Forced expiratory volume.
(3) Maximum expiratory flow rate.
(4) Maximum inspiratory flow rate.
(5) Lung compliance.
(6) Chest wall compliance.
(7) Airway resistance.

Lung volumes and capacities (Figure 4.1)

VC (Vital Capacity): maximum volume that can be expired follow-ing maximal inspiration.

IC (Inspiratory Capacity): volume that can be inspired from the resting end expiratory position.

IRV (Inspiratory Reserve Volume): volume that can be inspired from spontaneous end inspiratory position.

ERV (Expiratory Reserve Volume): volume that can be expired from spontaneous end expiratory position.

FRC (Functional Residual Capacity): volume in the lungs at the end of normal expiration.

RV (Residual Volume): volume in the lungs after maximal expir-ation.

TLC (Total Lung Capacity): volume in the lungs after maximal inspiration.

VT (Tidal Volume): volume of spontaneous breath.

Others: minute volume; respiratory dead space; alveolar ventilation.

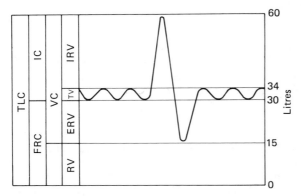

Figure 4.1 Repiratory functions: lung volumes in litres

Table 4.1 Range of normal values for lung volumes

	Vital capacity (l)	Residual volume (l)	Total lung capacity (l)
Age 20–39			
male	3.45–5.90	1.13–2.32	4.80–7.92
female	2.45–4.38	1.00–2.00	3.61–6.18
Age 40–59			
male	2.72–5.30	1.45–2.62	4.50–7.62
female	2.09–4.02	1.16–2.20	3.41–6.02
Age 60			
male	2.42–4.70	1.77–2.77	4.35–7.32
female	1.91–3.66	1.32–2.40	3.31–5.86

The range of normal values for lung volumes is shown in Table 4.1.

Diffusion and gas exchange

(1) Oxygen consumption.
(2) Diffusing capacity.
(3) Blood gases.

Pulmonary circulation

(1) Capillary blood flow.
(2) Pulmonary pressures.

Thoracic procedures

Sputum examination

Identifies infection and malignancy. Gram stain is a fundamental part of sputum investigation. For anaerobic infections, trans-tracheal aspiration is the best sampling technique.

Thoracocentesis

May be diagnosed or therapeutic. Previous chest X-rays PA and lateral are essential.

With the patient leaning forward, locally anaesthetized, sterilized and draped (Figure 4.2), the needle is passed over a rib (Figure 4.3). The fluid is sent for biochemistry, cultures, cell count and cytology.

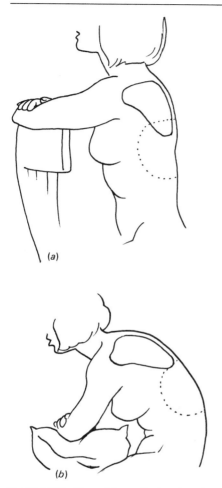

Figure 4.2 Position of the patient undergoing thoracocentesis

The actual tap can be done with needle, a small venous cannula or a trochar. Large or chronic pleural effusions drained too quickly may dispose to re-expansion pulmonary oedema.

Chest drainage

Pleural effusions, air, blood or pus may all require drainage with an indwelling tube.

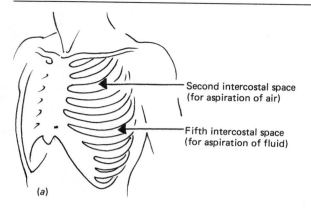

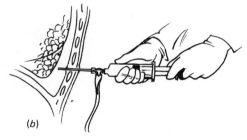

Figure 4.3 The pleural space is previously aspirated: (*a*) sites of aspiration; (*b*) catheter inserted into pleural space

Air is best evacuated through a high tube in the second space (mid-axillary line) or in the third space (anterior axillary line), the last being less painful, less muscular and less obtrusive. Fluid should be drained through the lowest point (usually seventh or eighth space in mid-axillary line). This should be checked by aspiration and sometimes by lipiodol contrast X-rays.

Lignocaine is infiltrated down the track above the rib. A skin incision is made and ligatures placed for tying the tube in and for closing the hole afterwards. The tube with its indwelling trochar and cannula is then thrust through the anaesthetized track above the rib. The tube is placed with its outermost hole within the pleura, preferably obliquely forwards away from the patient's weight-bearing back surfaces, and securely tied (Figures 4.4–4.6).

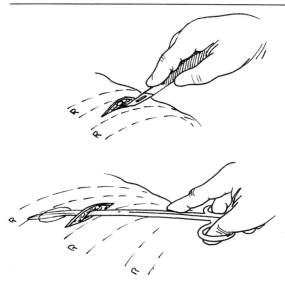

Figure 4.4 The skin is incised and the space above the incision is opened, trying to make a tunnel between the skin and the intercostal opening

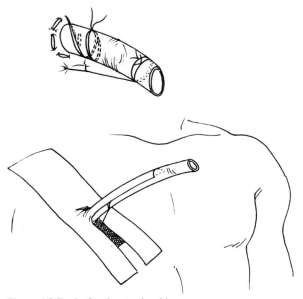

Figure 4.5 Drain fixation to the skin

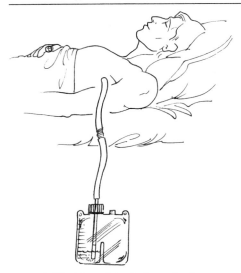

Figure 4.6 Position of the drainage bottle

Scalene node biopsy

Indications are enlarged palpable nodes in this region and staging of advanced pulmonary malignancy. The nodes commonly show lymphoma, tuberculosis, sarcoid or metastatic carcinoma. The right nodes are more commonly enlarged as they drain a greater area. In the chest only the left upper lobe drains into the left scalene nodes.

An incision is made above the clavicle, between the two borders of the sternomastoid. Lifting the omohyoid, the nodes are found on the scalene fascia.

Some structures to be avoided are the pleurae, local veins, transverse thoracic artery, phrenic nerve and thoracic duct.

Mediastinoscopy

Mediastinoscopy is used for the establishment of histology where enlarged mediastinal glands are found by X-rays or CT scans. The incision is made midway between the bottom of the sternal notch and the cricoid cartilage. Scissor dissection is made through the pretracheal fascia and then the finger is passed behind this fascial plane in front of the trachea (Figue 4.7).

The mediastinoscope can follow this track examining all tissues on the way. If there is any doubt before biopsy, a presumed lymph node can be distinguished from a vessel by prior needle aspiration.

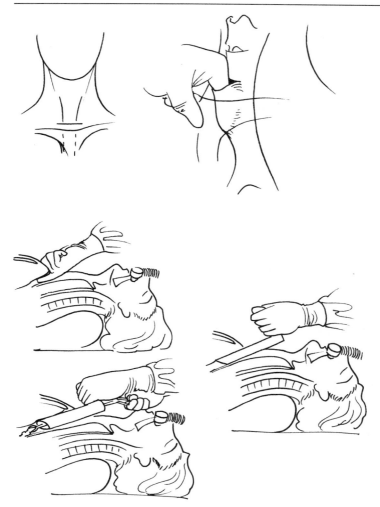

Figure 4.7 Mediastinoscopy: technique

Anterior mediastinotomy

Glands around the aortic arch to the left of the tracheal bifurcation are not accessible to mediastinoscopy. Similarly, anterior mediastinal glands on either side require this more anterior approach. Incision for 6–10 cm over the second cartilage (Figure 4.8), which is resected subperichondrially and the internal mammary artery

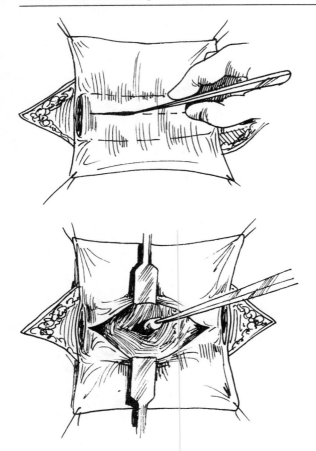

Figure 4.8 Mediastinotomy: technique

divided after ligation. The pleura can then frequently be swept laterally without penetration, giving access to the mediastinum. Careful haemostasis and avoidance of phrenic nerves are important.

Thoracoscopy

In the absence of pleural adhesions, nearly all parts of pleura can be viewed endoscopically by this method. The thoracoscope may be an adapted cytoscope, a bronchoscope or any other endoscope. Examination, biopsy, poudrage or other manoeuvres can thus be performed.

Pleural biopsy

The technique is as for thoracocentesis, but a cutting needle such as Cope's, Abrams or Tru-cut is used.

Lung biopsy

This can be bronchial, transtracheal, fine needle, Tru-cut and open. Fine needle biopsy has made accessible for histology peripheral lesions not reachable by bronchoscopy, such as localized infection in children and in immunocompromised patients, inoperable lesions and lesions in the apex. Tomograms and multiplane screening facilities are necessary.

Contraindications include bleeding tendency, multiple emphysematous bullae with poor lung function and circumstances more liable to provoke pneumothorax, haemoptysis or air embolus. Open lung biopsy may be necessary when transbronchial or percutaneous methods have failed.

Endotracheal intubation

Every doctor should be adept in this as apart from general anaesthesia and mechanical ventilation it may be necessary for removal of aspirated material, airway obstruction or trauma and similar life-threatening conditions.

A curved laryngoscope (McIntosh) is more common than a straight (Miller) one (Figure 4.9a and b). The tube size in general is 2–4 for infants, 4–7 for children and 7–10 for adults. The laryngoscope should display the vocal cords and the tube be inserted through them under direct vision. Laryngeal trauma, oesophageal intubation and over-inflation of the endotracheal tube balloon with subsequent mucosal damage and stenosis should be avoided.

Cricothyroidotomy

This includes the 'mini-tracheostomy'. A small cannula is introduced through the cricothyroid membrane (Figure 4.10) as an emergency for acute obstruction with difficult intubation, or electively for removal of sputum where tracheostomy is not thought to be necessary. Through this cannula secretions can be aspirated, oxygen administered, the bronchi washed and nebulized drugs given (Figure 4.11).

Patients known to have difficulty with sputum clearance, bad left

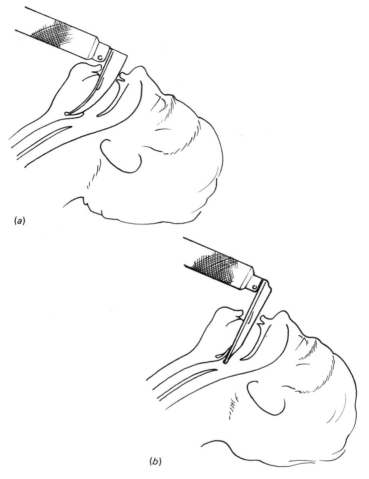

(a)

(b)

Figure 4.9 Endotracheal intubation with (a) a curved McIntosh laryngoscope and (b) a straight Miller laryngoscope

ventricular function, laryngeal incoordination or poor mental co-operation are potential candidates for this procedure.

If a proper tracheostomy is to be done, the mini-tracheostomy should not be employed. Of course, low tracheal obstruction is not helped by it.

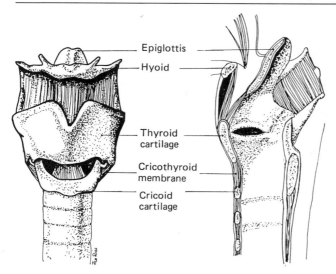

Figure 4.10 Laryngeal anatomy

Epiglottis

Hyoid

Thyroid cartilage

Cricothyroid membrane

Cricoid cartilage

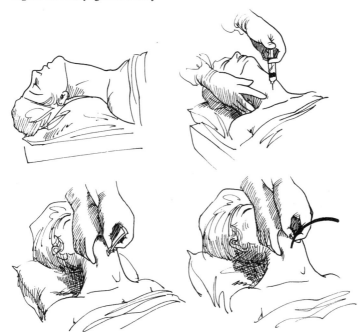

Figure 4.11 Mini-tracheostomy: technique

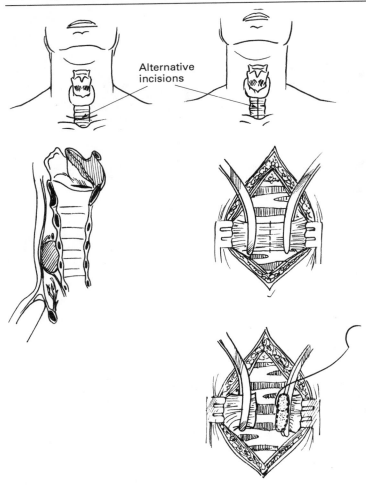

Figure 4.12 Tracheostomy: anatomical approach

Tracheostomy

This may be urgent (occlusion of the upper airway by trauma or diphtheria) or elective (in cases of prolonged intubation for ventilation or other purposes). The procedure is as for mediastinoscopy, making an incision midway between the cricoid cartilage and the bottom of the sternal notch, followed by scissor dissection of pretracheal fascia and the anterior surface of the trachea itself (Figure 4.12). Though the second and third ring the incision is made and it can be horizontal, vertical, inverted 'U' shaped or 'cross' shaped.

The most important aspect is the care of the tube, i.e. bronchial aspiration hourly; change of dressing daily; change of tube weekly.

Complications include: operative bleeding, pneumothorax, tracheo-oesophageal fistula, laryngeal nerve injury, paratracheal intubation, tube obstruction, aspiration, infection, tracheo-arterial fistula, stenosis, tracheomalacia, granuloma and permanent stoma. The pressure in the balloon should be sufficient to prevent excessive leakage from the ventilation circuit. High pressures may cause mucosal destruction with subsequent erosion and stricture.

Bronchoscopy (Figure 4.13)

This may be diagnostic or therapeutic, rigid or fibreoptic.

Indications

(1) Diagnostic: mainly to identify tumours, sites of haemoptysis, stenosis or rupture.
(2) Therapeutic: to evacuate foreign bodies or inhaled material including retained secretions after operations (causing atelectasis). Also in trauma to the airways and as a part of treatment in intrabronchial bleeding or bronchopleural fistula.

For therapeutic purposes the rigid bronchoscope gives better access. For diagnosis, the fibreoptic enables a better view of the upper lobes. Generally, rigid bronchoscopy is performed under general anaesthesia and fibreoptic under local. Abnormal coagulation, electrocardiographic or radiological hazards should be known about.

The patient should be starving, premedicated with atropine (0.6–1.2 mg i.v or i.m). Sedation is achieved with meperidine, pentobarbitone or diazepam for fibreoptic bronchoscopy. The pharynx is infiltrated with lignocaine.

Heavy bleeding may be controlled with a swab soaked in adrenaline, applied for 2–3 min. Massive bleeding may be treated by pressure with a swab, Fogarty catheter or Thompson bronchial blocker, fluid replacement and in some cases thoracotomy.

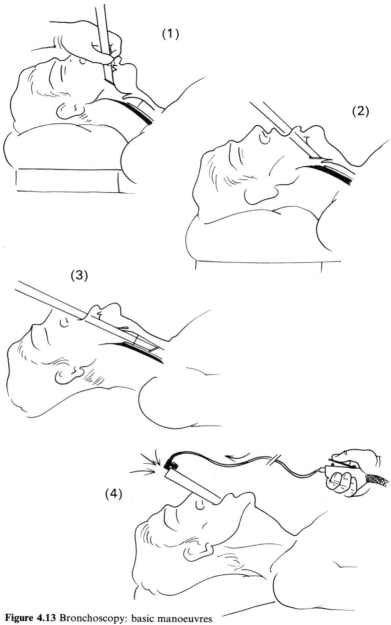

Figure 4.13 Bronchoscopy: basic manoeuvres

Respiratory failure

Defined in terms of arterial gases: breathing air at sea level the Pa_{O_2} is less than 60 mmHg (8 kPa). According to the Pa_{CO_2}, respiratory failure can be classified as:

Type I (Pa_{CO_2} below 50 mmHg or 6.7 kPa)
Type II (Pa_{CO_2} above 50 mmHg or 6.7 kPa)

Type I respiratory failure may be caused by uneven ventilation/ perfusion ratio, as occurs in chronic bronchitis and early emphysema, pneumonia, acute pulmonary oedema, pulmonary thromboembolism, collapse, fibrosing alveolitis, and other generalized pulmonary diseases. Treatment of this type of respiratory failure is based on high concentrations of inspired oxygen.

In Type II respiratory failure the mechanism of hyperventilation secondary to increased P_{CO_2} is inadequate, as can be seen in exacerbation or advanced phases of chronic bronchitis or emphysema, acute asthmatic attack, narcotic poisoning, neuromuscular disease and mechanical disorders of the thoracic cage. Treatment is with controlled oxygen adminstration in order to keep some hypoxaemic respiratory drive that prevents fatal respiratory acidosis. In severe cases mechanical ventilation is mandatory.

Adult respiratory distress syndrome

This is a non-specific type of respiratory failure, usually secondary to non-pulmonary disease, and characterized by increasing dyspnoea, severe hypoxaemia, lung infiltration clinically and on chest X-ray, and caused by disruption of the alveolar-capillary membrane with exudation of a fluid with high protein content into the interstitium and the alveoli.

There are many causes for it including trauma, sepsis, chemical pneumonitis and pancreatitis among others. The clinical course has been divided into four phases:

(1) Trauma, resuscitation and alkalosis secondary to the initial hyperventilation.
(2) Increased intrapulmonary shunt with hypoxaemia, high cardiac output, low P_{CO_2} and negative chest X-rays.
(3) Respiratory insufficiency refractory to oxygen administration and increased Pa_{CO_2}.
(4) Severe hypoxia and CO_2 retention with terminal failure.

Treatment should include fluid restriction, cardiac inotropic support, mechanical ventilation and treatment of complications.

Mechanical ventilation

Mechanical ventilation is indicated to improve alveolar ventilation and gas exchange where this fails in neurological disease, respiratory failure, muscular diseases, drug depression of nervous system, severe low cardiac output, and in the postoperative period to allow restoration of the patient's homeostasis.

Ventilation may be suggested by dyspnoea, the use of accessory muscles of ventilation, hypoxaemia, tachypnoea, V_D/V_T greater than 0.6, large alveolo-arterial gradient, a fall in residual functional capacity, alveolar collapse, increasing shunt and hypoxaemia.

Ventilatory modes are:

(1) *Controlled.* The ventilator is independent of the patient and does not respond to his ventilatory movements. It is indicated during surgery, in cases of central apnoea, and paralysis of spontaneous activity.
(2) *Assisted.* The ventilator is triggered by the patient's own respiratory effort.
(3) *Controlled/assisted.* The ventilator supports the patient's effort, adding an additional number of ventilatory excursions to avoid anoxia. Could be IMV (intermittent mandatory ventilation) or MMV (mandatory minute volume).
(4) *High frequency ventilation.* The rate is greater than 40/min with small tidal volumes. When given through a small orifice parallel with the airway and causing Venturi augmentation it is called high frequency jet ventilation (HFJV). The system in this case can be electromagnetic-pneumatic valve, fluidic, solenoid or flow interruptor. The other modality – high frequency oscillation (HFO) – gives a small volume and pulls it back and requires even lower pressures. Both types are indicated in barotrauma, bronchopleural fistula and neonatal respiratory failure.

Types of ventilators

The types of ventilators are:

(1) *Volume-cycled.* This delivers a preset volume each minute with resultant variations of pressure, e.g. Manley, Pulmovent, Ohio, Cape, Bennett MA2.
(2) *Pressure-cycled.* A predetermined pressure is given a certain number of times per minute, the volume varying according to the lung compliance, e.g. Bird ventilator.
(3) *Time-cycled.* The rate and duration of inspiration are preset, e.g. Servo, Servo 900B.

Each type has advantages and disadvantages. The volume-cycled ventilator may cause barotrauma by reaching excessive pressures to deliver a preset volume. The pressure-cycled, on the other hand, may deliver ineffective volumes where compliance is insufficient.

Monitoring during mechanical ventilation

Monitoring should include arterial pressure, heart rate, central venous pressure and, in critical cases, pulmonary wedge pressure and cardiac output. Mechanical ventilation affects the cardiac output and may damage the lung, elevating pulmonary resistance causing oedema and fibrosis. It can cause pulmonary infection, may cause hypocarbia and severe metabolic disturbances. High oxygen concentrations can lead to atelectasis, early fibrosis and neonatal eye damage (retrolental fibroplasia).

During mechanical ventilation the airway pressures and the intrapleural pressure are positive (as opposed to spontaneous ventilations) in inspiration. This decreases the right ventricular preload and may cause barotrauma.

Humidification of inspired gases is essential. The pressure in the balloon of the endotracheal tube must be just sufficient. Secretions should be aspirated frequently and the bacteriology of the sputum carefully monitored. Also, sedation should be given to avoid contests between the patient and the ventilator. Monitoring of ventilation must include frequent measurement of blood gases (automated blood gas analyser, continuous intra-arterial analyser, or continuous transcutaneous oxygen measurement). Tidal volume and minute volume can be controlled directly by true volume meters (intermittent as the wet spirometer, the bellow system, the piston system and the diaphragm system; or continuous as the gas meters and the Drager volumeters), and by flow meters (Wright respirometer, spiroflow, pneumotachograph, hot wire anemometer or ultrasound).

Discontinuation of ventilator

The patient is weaned from the ventilator when the original indications for mechanical ventilatory support are over and when the patient's reflexes, vital capacity, blood gases and chest X-rays show improvement once the F_{IO_2} is less than 50% and the IMV is used less than twice per minute. If the pH is normal, the P_{aCO_2} is < 50 mmHg (6.5 kPa), the P_{aO_2} is > 60–70 mmHg (8–9 kPa) with an F_{IO_2} of less than 40% and the ventilatory rate < 30/min, the patient is allowed to breathe room air through the tube and the arterial gases are measured afterwards. If the patient keeps the same levels after breathing room air and is not distressed or sleepy, extubation can proceed.

Patients in heart failure, very lethargic, with arrhythmias or low vital capacities (below 10 ml/kg) may require extra care over the course of extubation.

Alternatives to mechanical ventilation

Alternative ventilatory/respiratory aids such as CPAP through a face mask is occasionally helpful where endotracheal ventilation is not mandatory but early pulmonary oedema, small pulmonary contusions or broncho-aspirations exist.

Extreme respiratory failure despite maximum ventilatory support may be helped by extracorporeal membrane oxygenation (ECMO).

Pulmonary embolism

In this condition there may be pleuritic chest pain, dyspnoea, tachypnoea, augmented dead space, hypoxaemia, increased metabolic oxygen consumption, bronchoconstriction, alteration of coagulation systems, and any of the following haemodynamic changes:

- right ventricular overloading
- increased venous pressure
- displacement of the ventricular septum to the left
- release of catecholamines
- low cardiac output.

Ten per cent of patients die in the first hour, 30% of them without diagnosis. Many patients are asymptomatic and the only sign could be a cardiac arrhythmia. Investigations to prove the diagnosis are:

- blood gases (hypoxaemia)
- chest X-rays (possible hilar enlargement, pulmonary oligaemia, diaphragmatic elevation, pleural effusion, atelectasis)
- electrocardiogram (right axis, S_1-Q_3-T_3, right ventricular overload)
- radioactive lung scan (very accurate)
- pulmonary angiography (definitive diagnosis).

Prophylaxis

Avoidance of endothelial trauma and stagnation of blood flow, hence early mobilization of the lower limbs and low dose heparin after major surgical procedures to activate antithrombin 3 and block thromboplastin. Doses: 5000 units subcutaneously every 8–12 h.

Treatment (Figure 4.14)

(1) Well tolerated embolism: heparin 5000–10000 units i.v. loading dose, thereafter maintaining clotting time at 2–3 times normal. Warfarin instituted after 10 days and maintained for at least six months.
(2) Larger embolism with respiratory and cardiovascular embarrassment: thrombolytic therapy with urokinase or streptokinase.
(3) Massive embolism with life endangered: surgical embolectomy.

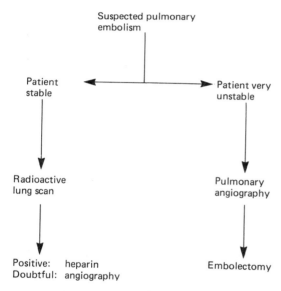

Figure 4.14 Scheme for management of suspected pulmonary embolism

Massive haemoptysis

When there is more than 500 ml of blood in 24 h or more than 200 ml of blood at any time inside the respiratory tree, the patient presents with acute respiratory failure and the diagnosis is massive haemoptysis.

As soon as diagnosed, the patient is placed in decubitus position with the affected side down. Immediate resuscitation with fluids, intubation if necessary, and proper diagnosis measures are started. Bronchoscopy is carried out as soon as possible using the rigid bronchoscope and, if difficult, the bleeding site is assessed with fibreoptic or lateral-viewed apparatus through the rigid tube. If there is a clear bleeding point, balloon occlusion may be performed using Fogarty or Foley catheter. Then operability is defined. The balloon could be left in place temporarily and bronchial artery embolization performed. If this is unsuccessful lobar or segmental resection may be necessary and should control the situation.

Pneumonia

The lung defends itself by coughing, ciliary action, mucus, lysozyme, lactoferrin, immunoglobulins (mainly A and G) and cellular response (macrophage, lymphocytic and neutrophilic).

Infection may occur by aspiration, colonization, inoculation and haematogenous spread. Aspiration is the most common. Inhalation spreads tuberculosis, *Legionella*, *Pneumococcus* and viruses; inoculation occurs in ventilator-transmitted pneumonia; colonization in elderly, immunosuppressed patients and nosocomial infection; and haematogenous infection results from endocarditis, pelvic thrombophlebitis, urinary sepsis and Gram-negative sepsis.

Pneumonia may be classified as:

(1) *Atypical*, e.g. *Mycoplasma, Legionella*, tubercle bacilli, fungus and viruses.

(2) *Community acquired*. In younger people: *Streptococcus pneumoniae* and *Mycoplasma*. In older people: *Streptococcus pneumoniae, Haemophilus influenzae*, enterobacteria and *Staphylococcus aureus*.

(3) *Hospital acquired*, e.g. *Klebsiella, Pseudomonas, Staphylococcus* and enterobacteria.

(4) *Immunosuppressed patients*, i.e. terminally ill, elderly, chronic systemic diseases, malnourishment, diabetes, AIDS, alcoholism and therapeutic immunosuppression as well as cancer. Organisms are: bacterial (5–25%); fungal (10–30%); viral (2–4%); *Pneumocystis* (10–40%) and indeterminate (25–40%). Also, pneumonia may be non-infectious in 15% of cases.

Sputum is necessary for bacteriological confirmation and it may be obtained by expectoration, transtracheal aspiration or by bronchoscopy (with or without bronchial lavage). Biopsy may be needed. Treatment of ventilatory problems, malnutrition, dehydration and associated problems and complications are as important as antibiotics. While awaiting full culture and sensitivity, some form of treatment is started based on the Gram stain.

- Gram-positive cocci in pairs (*Streptococcus*): penicillin or erythromycin.
- Gram-positive cocci (*Staph. aureus*): a cephalosporin, vancomycin.
- Gram-negative coccobacilli (*H. influenzae*): a cephalosporin, cotrimoxazole, chloramphenicol.
- Gram-negative bacilli (*Klebsiella*): a cephalosporin plus an aminoglycoside.
- If no organisms seen (unusual pathology): erythromycin.
- If no Gram stain available:
  * Young patient in good condition: erythromycin.
  * Young patient debilitated: a cephalosporin.
  * Elderly patient: a cephalosporin/co-trimoxazole.
  * Immunocompromised patient: a cephalosporin plus an aminoglycoside.
  * AIDS: erythromycin/co-trimoxazole.

Acute emergencies in asthma

Widespread airway obstruction due to periodic and generally reversible contraction of smooth muscle of the respiratory tract.

Asthma can be extrinsic (allergy), intrinsic (non-identifiable cause), drug-induced, exercise-induced and occupational. During the acute episode there is wheezing, low blood pressure, severe dyspnoea, low P_{CO_2} and alkalosis.

The main differential diagnosis is with foreign bodies, pulmonary oedema, pulmonary thromboembolism, atelectasis and pneumothorax.

Drug treatment

Treatment is based initially on beta agonists, xanthines and oxygen, followed by steroids if no good response is obtained and by ventilatory support in life-threatening cases.

Beta agonists increase cyclic AMP in the smooth muscle cells of the airways. They are:
- Isoprenaline (sublingually 10–20 mg; inhalation 80–240 µg/dose no more than 8 times in 24 h).
- Albuterol (i.v. or inhaled).

- Epinephrine (0.3 mg subcutaneously every 20 min).
- Terbutaline (0.25–0.5 mg subcutaneously).

Xanthine derivatives are:

- Theophylline (60–250 mg 3–4 times daily in adults).
- Aminophylline (6 mg/kg i.v. loading dose over 20 min; infusion: 0.1–0.5 mg/kg/h)

Corticosteroids are represented by hydrocortisone (3 mg/kg every 6 h). Afterwards it can be switched to prednisolone (40–60 mg/day) reducing progressively. Steroids increase the response of smooth muscle to cyclic AMP. Atropine, which lowers the content of cyclic guanosine monophosphate, can be administered nebulized at 0.05 mg/kg in saline solution.

Indications for ventilation are respiratory arrest, progressive CO_2 increase with respiratory acidosis and severe clinical deterioration. In particular cases general anaesthesia has been used (halothane) as well as bronchoscopy and bronchial lavage.

Abbreviations in respiratory medicine

a	arterial blood
A	alveolar gas
B	barometric
BP	barometric pressure
c	capillary blood
C	gas concentration in blood phase
D	dead space gas
D	diffusing capacity
Do_2	oxygen diffusing capacity
$D\dot{V}$	gas volume/unit time
E	expired gas
f	respiratory frequency
F	fractional gas concentration
Fio_2	fractional O_2 concentration in inspired gas
I	inspired gas
P	gas pressure
$\bar{P}$	mean gas pressure
$\bar{P}ao_2$	mean arterial O_2 pressure
Q	volume of blood
$\dot{Q}$	volume of blood/unit time
R	respiratory exchange ratio

S	haemoglobin saturation
So_2	oxygen haemoglobin saturation
T	tidal gas
v	venous blood
V	gas volume
V_A	volume alveolar gas
$\dot{V}_A$	alveolar ventilation
V_D	dead space gas volume
V_{O_2}	oxygen consumption
V_T	tidal volume

Tables of normal values

Table 4.2 Respiratory indices (adult 60–70 kg)

Lung weight	800 g
Number of alveoli	296×10^6
Pulmonary capillary flow	5400 ml/min
Pulmonary capillary volume	60 ml
Respiratory rate	12–14/min
Dead space	150 ml (2.2 ml/kg)
Alveolar ventilation	4.2 litres/min
Tidal volume	400–600 ml
Minute volume	5–6 litres/min
Total lung capacity	5.0–6.5 litres
Inspiratory reserve volume	3.30–3.75 litres
Expiratory reserve volume	0.95–1.20 litres
Functional residual capacity	2.3–2.8 litres
Residual volume	1.2–1.7 litres
Inspiratory capacity	3.6–4.3 litres
Vital capacity	4.2–4.8 litres
Forced expiratory volume in 1 s (FEV_1)	75% of VC
Peak expiratory flow rate	400 litres/min
Peak inspiratory flow rate	300 litres/min
Maximum ventilatory volume	120 litres/min
CO_2 diffusing capacity	17–20 ml/min/mmHg
Total lung and chest wall compliance	0.1 litres/cmH$_2$O
Chest wall compliance	0.2 litres/cmH$_2$O

Table 4.3 Gases (at BP 760 mmHg or 101.1 kPa)

Inspired air
P_{O_2}	158 mmHg or 21.06 kPa
P_{CO_2}	0.3 mmHg or 0.04 kPa
P_{N_2}	596 mmHg or 79.46 kPa
P_{H_2O}	5 mmHg or 0.67 kPa

Expired air
P_{O_2}	116 mmHg or 15.47 kPa
P_{CO_2}	28 mmHg or 3.73 kPa
P_{N_2}	568 mmHg or 75.73 kPa
P_{H_2O}	47 mmHg or 6.27 kPa

Alveolar gas
P_{AO_2}	103 mmHg or 13.73 kPa
P_{ACO_2}	40 mmHg or 5.33 kPa
P_{AN_2}	570 mmHg or 75.99 kPa
P_{H_2O}	47 mmHg or 6.27 kPa

Mixed venous blood
P_{VO_2}	37–42 mmHg or 4.93–5.60 kPa
P_{VCO_2}	40–52 mmHg or 5.33–6.93 kPa
P_{VN_2}	573 mmHg or 76.39 kPa
pH	7.32–7.42

Arterial blood
P_{aO_2}	90–110 mmHg or 12.00–14.67 kPa
P_{aCO_2}	34–46 mmHg or 4.53–6.13 kPa
P_{aN_2}	573 mmHg or 76.39 kPa
pH	7.36–7.44

Thoracic Surgery

Spontaneous pneumothorax

This is the presence of air in the pleural cavity not caused by trauma. It is accepted that the quality of collagen is defective in many of these patients. It is called primary when presenting in previously healthy people and secondary when diagnosed in patients with pulmonary disease (chronic obstructive airway disease being the most common).

The management is summarized in Figure 5.1.

Cardiothoracic trauma

Trauma in some countries is the third most common cause of death, and cardiothoracic trauma is present in 50% of deaths due to trauma. When located to the thorax only, the mortality is about 5%; when there is another system compromised mortality raises to 15%; when trauma affects more than one organ or system, mortality is 30%

The intial management includes adequate airway, vital observations, external bleeding control and complete clinical examination. Also, insertion of at least two intravenous lines, immobilization of the neck and prompt fluid replacement.

The location of the site of impact helps in the investigations of associated lesions. Upper thoracic trauma implies higher incidence of lesions in the base of the neck, mainly laryngotracheal and pharyngo-oesophageal. Middle thoracic trauma goes with damage to mediastinal, spinal and neurological structures. Lower thoracic trauma frequently compromises abdominal viscera, especially liver, spleen and pancreas. X-ray facilities should be available, as well as all the equipment necessary ready for an emergency thoracotomy in theatre or in the emergency room. Nevertheless, even with all these resources, 30% of deaths due to thoracic trauma occur in hospital.

Thoracic lesions can be easily classified into three groups:

127

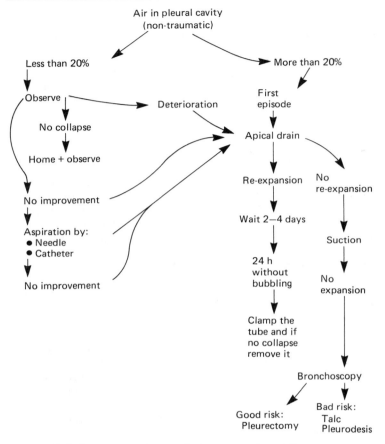

Figure 5.1 Scheme for management of spontaneous pneumothorax

(1) Rapidly lethal lesions, i.e. lesions that could kill the patient in a matter of minutes:
    (a) airway obstruction;
    (b) tension pneumothorax;
    (c) open pneumothorax;
    (d) massive haemothorax;
    (e) flail chest;
    (f) cardiac tamponade.
(2) Potentially lethal lesions, i.e. lesions that can kill the patient in a matter of hours:

(a) pulmonary contusion;
(b) aortic rupture;
(c) tracheobronchial rupture;
(d) oesophageal rupture;
(e) diaphragmatic rupture;
(f) myocardial contusion.
(3) Non immediately life threatening lesions:
(a) single haemothorax;
(b) single pneumothorax;
(c) rib fractures;
(d) sternal fractures;
(e) soft tissue lesions;
(f) traumatic chylothorax;
(g) intrathoracic foreign bodies;
(h) subcutaneous emphysema;
(i) others.

Rapidly lethal lesions (Figure 5.2)

Airway obstruction (Figure 5.2a)

Note patency of nose and mouth, intercostal retraction, quality of respiratory movements and obvious signs of respiratory distress.

Extract foreign bodies from the mouth and lift the jaws, provided that there is no cervical fracture, to keep the airway free from obstruction. If the patient is unconscious, an oral airway should be inserted. If there is respiratory insufficiency, intubate.

Tension pneumothorax (Figure 5.2c)

Pulmonary collapse, shifting of the mediastinum to the contralateral side, lowering of venous return and severe haemodynamic compromise are all indications of this condition. Clinically, respiratory distress, lack of ventilatory movements, cyanosis, distant cardiac sounds and bulky hemithorax indicate increased intrathoracic tension.

Treatment is the immediate drainage of air.

Open pneumothorax (Figure 5.2e)

'Pendeluft' increases effective dead space. Limited ventilatory capacity, lowered venous return and mediastinal movement cause haemodynamic deterioration.

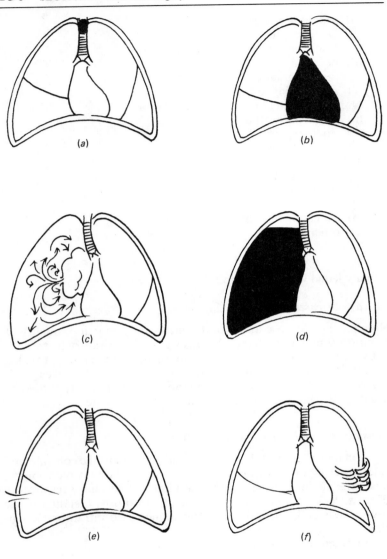

Figure 5.2 Rapidly lethal lesions: (*a* airway obstruction; (*b*) cardiac tamponade; (*c*) tension pneumothorax; (*d*) massive haemothorax; (*e*) open pneumothorax; (*f*) flail chest

Massive haemothorax (Figure 5.2*d*)

More than 2000 ml of blood in the pleural cavity. Mortality rate is 4% when it is associated with penetrating trauma and nearly 50% when the cause is blunt trauma. It usually presents with hypovolaemic shock, severe hypoventilation and clinical signs of pleural effusion. One litre of blood is the minimum perceptible in the supine chest X-ray.

Treatment includes fluid infusion, blood transfusion, thoracic drainage and thoracotomy when indicated. The indications for surgery are:

- deep shock
- more than 2000 ml of blood collected within the first 4 h after trauma
- more than 200 ml of blood through the thoracic drain every hour for four consecutive hours
- more than 400 ml of blood in any hour.

Flail chest (Figure 5.2*f*)

A segment of chest wall in anatomical and functional discontinuity with the rest of the thoracic cage because of multiple fractures restricts pulmonary parenchyma, increases ventilatory work, diminishes tidal volume and oxygen transport, and increases the dead space.

The initial treatment is pressure to stop paradoxical movement. Oxygen and aggressive analgesia may obviate ventilatory support. Mechanical ventilation may become necessary if there is need of general anaesthesia for other reasons, associated pulmonary contusion, central nervous system trauma and signs of progressive respiratory failure. Where prolonged ventilation is poorly supervised, surgical fixation of the flail segment may enable the patient to be nursed successfully in normal wards.

Cardiac tamponade (Figure 5.2*b*)

In blunt trauma, cardiac tamponade is generally lethal. In penetrating trauma a cardiac wound must be suspected in any epigastric or parasternal wound.

The clinical picture includes distant heart sounds, high venous pressure and hypotension. In some cases the patient is in deep shock and a paradoxical pulse can be detected. In some doubtful cases, if the patient is stable enough, fluoroscopy or echocardiography may demonstrate the intrapericardial fluid.

Sometimes pericardiocentesis can be used, but this may be a

temporary measure to avoid severe haemodynamic compromise in the emergency room until the patient has a definitive operation.

Potentially lethal lesions (Figure 5.3)

Pulmonary contusion

Mainly related to blunt trauma when the glottis is closed. The seriousness varies from the small lung haematoma to the so called 'traumatic lung' that usually appears after the initial trauma. What really impairs the prognosis in these patients is fluid overloading. Therefore, intravenous fluids should be limited up to 1000 ml in the initial resuscitation and to 30 ml/kg/day for the next 72 h (provided there is not any associated lesion that requires different treatment). Also, frusemide, analgesia, physiotherapy and methylprednisolone are part of the management.

Aortic rupture

Just 15% of these patients reach the hospital. Subtotal rupture at the left subclavian artery level is the most common situation. A high speed blunt injury in a young patient with chest X-ray with signs of widening of the upper mediastinum, possible deviation of the left main bronchus and tracheal bifurcation, supraclavicular opacity, obliteration of the normal cardiac contour should indicate an aortogram and prompt surgical repair or replacement of the damaged segment, usually the isthmus of the aorta.

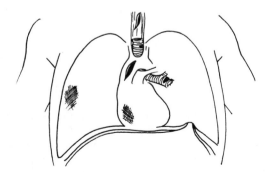

Figure 5.3 Potentially lethal lesions

Tracheobronchial rupture

This results from tracheal compression against the spine, distension of the airways with closed glottis and hyperextension of the bronchial tree. Fractures of the larynx produce dysphonia and subcutaneous emphysema. The majority of lesions of the bronchi occur at 2.5 cm from the carina, and the clinical picture depends on the degree of communication between the ruptured segment and the pleural space. Pneumothorax refractory to conventional treatment, pneumomediastinum, haemoptysis and signs of respiratory failure can be present. There may be linear tears or complete transection and crushing. Bronchoscopic diagnosis should be followed by surgical repair. Cardiopulmonary bypass may be helpful when both main bronchi are transected.

Oesophageal rupture

Epigastric trauma may rupture the lower third of the oesophagus. Vomiting against a closed glottis of an overfilled stomach may split the oesophagus from top to bottom (Boerhaave). In both situations there is upper abdominal pain, cervical emphysema, dysphagia and sometimes gastrointestinal bleeding and early sepsis due to mediastinitis.

A contrast swallow with hydrosoluble medium and, in some cases, oesophagoscopy confirm the diagnosis. The treatment is surgical and, depending on the time elapsed, primary suture, oesophageal exclusion or oesophageal resection may be performed.

Diaphragmatic rupture

This is more frequent on the left side. The clinical picture may range from local absence of symptoms to different degrees of shock. There is abdominal pain, hypotension and chest X-rays show diaphragmatic elevation, gas of an abnormal pattern within the chest and displacement of a nasogastric tube. The spleen may be visible above the diaphragm. Treatment is surgical.

Myocardial contusion

This occurs in at least 20% of severe thoracic trauma. The surgical pathology and the clinical picture is that of myocardial ischaemia as is the treatment, consisting of close monitoring and arrhythmia control as well as inprovement of low cardiac output.

Non immediately life threatening lesions (Figure 5.4)

These include well tolerated degrees of haemothorax, pneumo-thorax, soft tissue injuries, intrathoracic foreign bodies and bone fractures. Special considerations should be given to the so-called 'single rib fractures' which can be very dangerous if overlooked. They are frequently associated with pulmonary contusion and the pain may impair ventilatory mechanics. The mortality rate in single rib fractures in patients over 80 years is about 20%.

Patients at risk are the elderly, chronic respiratory patients and those with an associated pleural effusion. Treatment is local anaesthetic blockage with lignocaine 1%.

Injuries to the first and second ribs, as well as scapular and sternal fractures, might be associated with severe intrathoracic injuries.

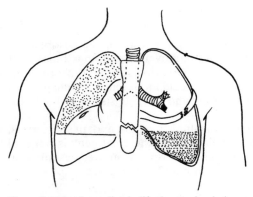

Figure 5.4 Non immediately life threatening lesions

Lung abscess

This is a necrotic, often encapsulated and cavitated mass of infected lung tissue. Important causes are:

(1) Aspiration (general anaesthesia, alcoholism, central nervous system injuries and general debilitation). The main microorganisms are anaerobic: *Bacteroides fragilis, Fusobacterium nuclea-tum*, etc.
(2) Postpneumonic (alcoholics, immunosuppressed, diabetics, cancer patients, renal failure and transplantation). Specific causes are: *Klebsiella pneumoniae, Pseudomonas, Staphylococcus aureus* and *Streptococcus*. Sometimes there is no specific cause.

(3) Secondary to regional or distant sepsis (carcinoma, sequestration, broncho-oesophageal fistulae, foreign bodies, pulmonary infarction).

The clinical presentation is often with foul sputum, radiologically localized opacities, cavitation, necrotizing pneumonia and pyopneumothorax. Bacteriology is obtained from sputum, transtracheal or percutaneous needle aspiration.

Management is based on antibiotics, pus evacuation, and drainage; resection of necrotic tissues only if necessary. First line antibiotics are penicillin G, metronidazole and cephalosporins. Thereafter, according to bacteriological advice.

Drainage can be performed by bronchoscopy, or externally when the lung is thoroughly adherent to the pleura. A tube suffices if the pus is thin, but it may need to be open drainage with very thick pus. Pulmonary resection is required if there is associated malignancy.

Secondary complications such as emphyema or bronchopleural fistula are treated on their merits.

Bronchiectasis

This consists of permanent dilatation of the bronchi, primary or secondary to inflammatory or obstructive disease, that destroys muscle and elastic tissue, replacing them with fibrosis and causing lung damage.

Congenital causes are congenital cystic disease, alpha and gamma globulin deficiencies, alpha-1 antitrypsin deficiency and Kartagener syndrome. Acquired causes are mainly related to obstruction with mucus stasis and infection causing dilatation and destruction of bronchial wall.

Clinically it presents as chronic respiratory disease with cough, fetid sputum, finger clubbing and general debility. Complications may be the first sign: suppurative brain disease, lung abscess, empyema or widespread sepsis. Bronchoscopy reveals pus in dilated bronchi. Bronchography, the definitive diagnostic measure, shows the dilated bronchi.

Treatment is medical with postural drainage, assisted coughing, antibiotics and aerosol bronchial dilators, mucolytics and cough stimulants. Surgery is indicated only when these measures fail in very symptomatic patients with abundant purulent sputum, haemoptysis and recurrent infections. It should be avoided in patients younger than two years and in high risk old patients with diffuse disease, established pulmonary hypertension and when bronchiectasis is part of systemic non-correctable disease. Resection should be adequate but not excessive since recurrence is possible.

Empyema thoracis

Empyema is the accumulation of pus in a natural cavity. In the pleura it usually has three phases:

(1) Exudative, with thin fluid, low cellular content and frequently negative culture.
(2) Fibrinopurulent, with fibrin, polymorphonuclear cells and more viscous fluid.
(3) Organizing, with thick fluid, pus and fibroblasts.

Later still the empyema may point through the chest wall as 'empyema necessitans', and there may be loculation trapping the lung.

The aetiology can be:

(1) Postinfection (pneumonia, oesophageal perforation, peritonitis, subphrenic abscess, mediastinitis).
(2) Postoperative (pneumonectomy, lobectomy, oesophagectomy, thoracotomy).
(3) Post-traumatic (including iatrogenic oesophageal perforations).

Bacteriology may show anaerobic bacteria, Gram negatives, *Staphylococcus*, *Streptococcus* and opportunistic infections in immunodepressed patients.

The diagnosis is confirmed by chest X-rays and thoracocentesis.

Empyema management (Figure 5.5) must include antibiotic treatment, drainage of pus, lung re-expansion, treatment of primary causes, respiratory support if necessary, nutritional care and treatment of complications. Surgical options available are tube thoracostomy, open thoracostomy, decortication, muscle transplants, space sterilization and thoracoplasty.

Septic shock

Septic shock is an extremely serious condition where disseminated infection leads to a severe perfusion deficit and cellular metabolic insufficiency. Despite the advent of new antibiotics and more aggressive treatment, septic shock carries 50% mortality.

There is release of mediators like ELM (endogenous leucocyte mediator), EP (endogenous pyrogen) and LAF (lymphocyte activa-

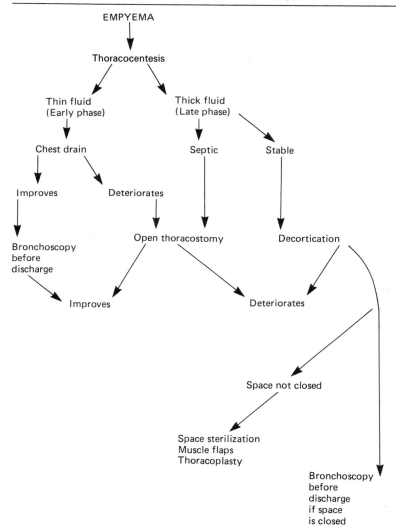

Figure 5.5 Scheme for management of empyema

tor factor) which bring about a rise in protein catabolism, hormones (insulin, glucagon), and other substances such as endorphins. At the cellular level there is increased lymphoycte production, macrophage activity and phagocytosis. Vasodilatation, increase in vascular permeability, activation of plasminogen, fibrin degradation and kallikrein stimulation impair cardiovascular competence. Traditionally, septic shock has been classified into two groups:

(1) *Low resistance septic shock* – with hypotension, low peripheral vascular tone, increased cardiac output and increased peripheral circulation.

(2) *High resistance septic shock* – a more advanced phase of the previous one with poor tissue oxygenation, very low blood pressure and increased peripheral vascular resistance. The cardiac output is progressively low. A catabolic state ensues from tissue inefficiency.

Preventive measures are vastly more important than treatment of septic shock, especially the avoidance of cross infection, simply by washing hands before any procedure and after examining any patient.

Once diagnosed, the source of sepsis must be removed and the patient fully covered with appropriate antibiotics. Severe sepsis creates metabolic problems and a complete regimen of nutrition should be given to avoid the consequences of catabolism.

Multisystem failure in surgical patients

Major surgery or trauma, sepsis, massive blood loss, old age and severe underlying disease cause multiple organ failure. The inadequate perfusion of body cells caused by hypovolaemia and sepsis, respiratory failure and severe malnutrition are associated with multisystem failure.

Renal failure: less than 100 ml of urine in 24 h or failure to concentrate with raised serum creatinine.

Hepatic failure: raised bilirubin, LDH, SGOT, SGPT and altered clotting.

Gastrointestinal failure: usually active gastrointestinal bleeding or pancreatitis.

Coagulation system failure: more than 25% increase in various coagulation times or less than 100 000 platelets/ml.

Multisystem failure exists if two or more organs are failing.

Foreign bodies in airways

In adults the main cause is food; in children it is food, peanuts and plastic objects.

A Heimlich manoeuvre should be first attempted. If unsuccessful and main airway obstruction continues, do cricothyroidotomy or emergency tracheostomy in extreme cases. If time is available, laryngoscopy and bronchoscopy will help to take the foreign body out.

Vomiting and aspiration cause particularly severe problems from chemical reaction and superinfection. This situation is common in alcoholics, after seizures and in neurological problems, as well as in any type of cardiac arrest. Treatment should include antibiotics, steroids, bronchoscopy and lavage, oxygen, bronchodilators and proper cultures.

Drowning may be dry (due to reflex closure of glottis due to submersion and bronchospasm) or wet. The latter could be due to sea water, which is hyperosmolar to serum, causing pulmonary oedema by osmotic mechanisms, hypovolaemia and lethargy (as magnesium content is high in sea water). Fresh water, on the other hand, passes through the alveolocapillary membrane causing haemolysis, hyponatraemia and fluid overloading if the patient survives the acute episode of hypoxia. Also, the dropping in surfactant causes atelectasis and hypoxia.

Lung cancer

Victims usually smoke heavily. Symptomatology is wide: dyspnoea, cough, haemoptysis, pleuritic pain, clubbing, bone pain, dysphagia, cervical nodes, hepatic symptoms and neuroendocrine symptoms amongst others.

Primary types are: squamous (30–35%); undifferentiated including small-cell, large-cell and oat-cell tumour (25%); adenocarcinoma (5–15%); and uncommonly bronchoalveolar tumours. Metastatic tumours are also common in the lung.

Investigation must define histological type of tumour, extension and operability, and should include chest X-ray, sputum cytology, bronchoscopy with brushings, washings or biopsy, CT scan, mediastinoscopy or mediastinotomy, scans of liver, bone and brain, and lung function tests to assess how well a patient would tolerate removal of pulmonary tissue.

Operation is usually for the improvement of patient's long-term prognosis, rather than the alleviation of symptoms and is therefore undertaken only when total resection is probable. The exception to this is potential or actual Pancoast tumour.

   Relative contraindications are: intrathoracic extension with pericardial, oesophageal, pleural, mediastinal, phrenic nerve paralysis, and rib extension. Absolute contraindications are: caval involvement, distant metastases and recurrent nerve involvement. Nevertheless, when the tumour involves the heart, great vessels, trachea, oesophagus, vertebral body or produces pleural effusion, it is automatically classified as T3 and is at least Stage IIIb.

TNM classification

T (Tumour)

Tx = malignant cells present. X-rays and bronchoscopy negative.
T0 = no evidence of primary tumour. This is the category where only metastases are found.
T1 = tumour < 3 cm. No invasion of lobar bronchus.
T2 = tumour > 3 cm, or invading visceral pleura, obstructing a bronchus, or extending to hilar region, bronchoscopy shows tumour confined to bronchus or more than 2 cm from the carina, and pulmonary obstructive complications involving less than entire lung.
T3 = tumour extending into chest wall, diaphragm, mediastinum or pericardium, not involving heart, great vessels, trachea, oesophagus or vertebral body. Tumour in main bronchus < 2 cm from carina, not involving carina.
T4 = tumour invading mediastinum, heart, great vessels, trachea, oesophagus, vertebral body or carina, or producing malignant pleural effusion.

N (Nodes) – Figure 5.6

N0 = no demonstrable metastases to nodes.
N1 = metastasis to lymph nodes in peribronchial or ipsilateral region, including direct extension.
N2 = metastasis to ipsilateral mediastinal lymph nodes or subcarinal lymph nodes.
N3 = metastasis to contralateral, mediastinal, hilar, scalene or supraclavicular lymph nodes.

M (Metastases)

M0 = no known distant metastases.
M1 = positive distant metastases.

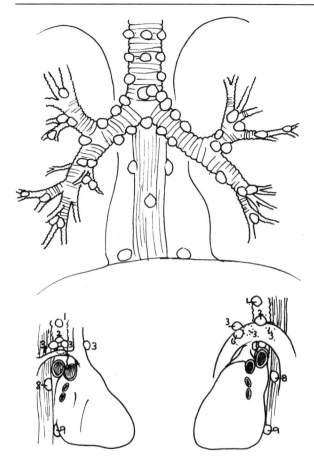

Figure 5.6 Node stations of the lungs and bronchi

Staging

CT scan and magnetic resonance imaging (MRI) scan as staging procedures

CT scan is very sensitive for hilar and mediastinal nodal enlargement (nodes < 1 cm in diameter are only 3% likely to be malignant; between 1 and 2 cm this likelihood is 36%; > 2 cm is 93%). CT scan is also sensitive to chest wall invasion.

MRI differentiates well between malignant and benign nodes.

Table 5.1

Occult	Tx N0 M0
Stage 0	T1S (Carcinoma *in situ*)
Stage I	TI N0 M0; T2 N0 M0
Stage II	T1 N1 M0; T2 N1 M0
Stage IIIa	T3 N0 M0; T3 N1 M0; T1 N2 M0
	T2 N2 M0; T3 N2 M0
Stage IIIb	T1 N3 M0; T2 N3 M0; T3 N3 M0;
	T4 N3 M0; T4 N0 M0; T4 N1 M0;
	T4 N2 M0; T4 N3 M0
	Thus: Any T4, any N3, always M0
Stage IV	Any T, any N, M1

There is a 23% false positive rate in non-invasive evaluation of the mediastinum, thus chest X-rays (if doubtful) should be followed by CT scan. If this, or a definitive chest X-ray shows involved mediastinal glands, these should be assessed and biopsied if < 2 cm; if negative, thoracotomy should be carried out.

Likely outcome

Out of 100 patients, 50 are likely to be definitively inoperable, 10% found inoperable at thoracotomy, and 40% having resection. From all resected specimens half will show incomplete resection and the other half (just 20% of the total) will have resection with hope of cure.

Although surgery is the most desirable treatment, inoperability must be rigidly excluded. After resection survival is 60% in Stage I, 30% in Stage II and just 10% in Stage III.

Radiotherapy may be employed for squamous or undifferentiated tumours which are inoperable, recurrent, advanced, or where operation is contraindicated. Radiotherapy may be employed pre-operatively for Pancoast tumour or postoperatively where histology of the operative specimen shows possible tumour outside the boundaries of surgery.

Some Stage III patients may benefit from surgery. T3 N0 patients have 30–50% five-year survival after resection; T3 N1 will have in some series 15–20% five-year survival; and T3 N2 between 5 and 10%. Resection may include chest wall, mediastinal tissue, diaphragm and atrial wall, and for Pancoast tumour some ribs and tissue around the root of the neck.

Small-cell carcinoma is rarely a surgical condition and is a systemic disease from its early stages.

Metastatic tumours may be resected even if multiple, provided that the primary tumour has been adequately controlled and the patient is healthy. The tumour should be resected with more than 1 cm clearance. Breast and epidermoid carcinomas do worst after resection of pulmonary metastases and urinary tract and testicular tumours do the best. Sarcomas are in between.

Benign tumours of the lung are not very common. They are usually asymptomatic and picked up on routine X-rays. Treatment of the most common lesion (hamartoma) is observation or conservative resection. Epithelial papillomas and polyps are treated by endoscopic resection. Vascular tumours are usually treated by irradiation (haemangioma), resection (lymphangioma), lobectomy or embolization (AV fistula). Fibromatous chondromas and adenomas are generally treated by lobar resection.

Thoracotomy

Some anatomical and surgical details of thoracotomy are illustrated in Figures 5.7–5.12.

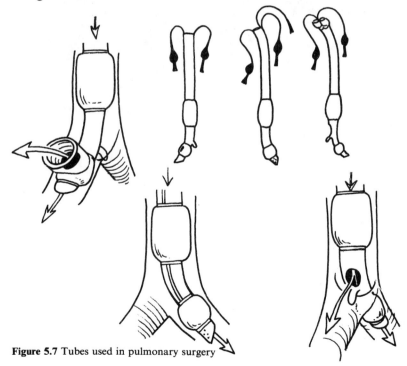

Figure 5.7 Tubes used in pulmonary surgery

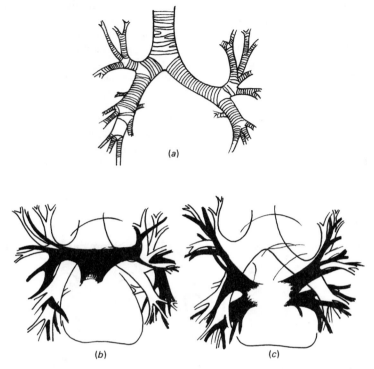

(a)

(b)   (c)

Figure 5.8 Normal anatomy of (a) bronchial, (b) arterial and (c) venous pulmonary systems

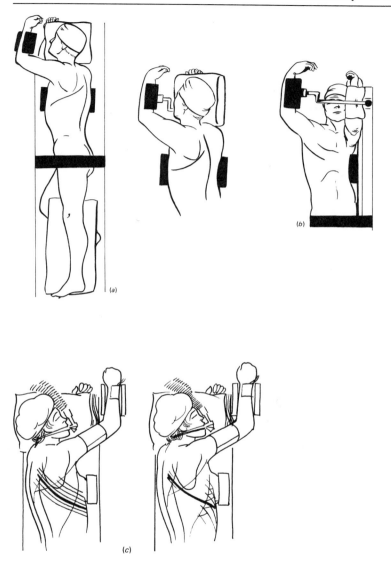

Figure 5.9 Position of the patient for thoracotomy: (a) posterolateral view;
(b) frontal view; (c) muscular incisions in posterolateral thoracotomy

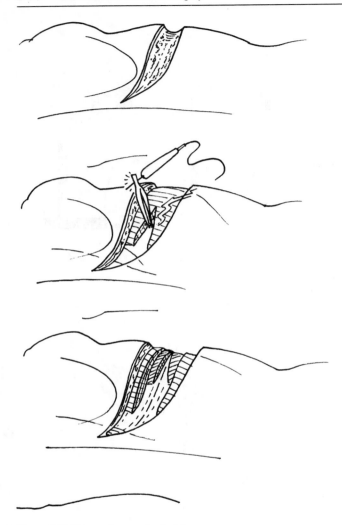

Figure 5.10 Skin and muscular incisions

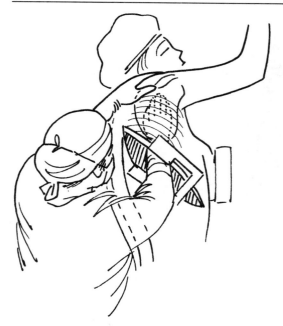

Figure 5.11 The surgeon counting ribs

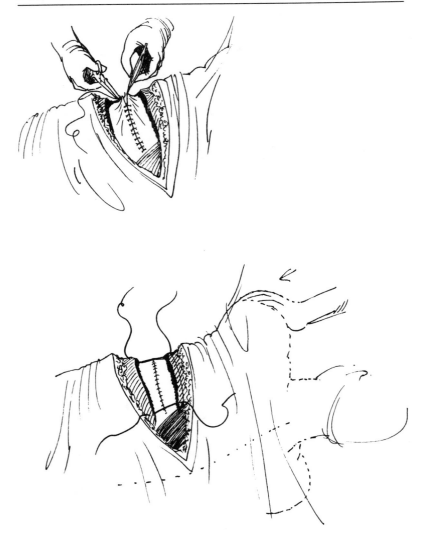

Figure 5.12 Closing the chest

Pulmonary resection

Right upper lobectomy

(1) From the front clean anterior pulmonary hilus between the phrenic nerve and the lung, from the bottom of the superior pulmonary vein between the azygos vein and the bronchus, then down the back of the hilus past the upper lobe bronchus take-off.

(2) Isolate anterior trunk of pulmonary artery by retracting the apical vein and divide it.

(3) For upper lobe division of superior pulmonary vein: take either apical vein, posterior vein, anterior vein or all at once if certain that the middle lobe vein is safe and avoiding penetration of the posterior vein in an attempt to get all together.

(4) Next, clean the interlobar segment of the pulmonary artery, visualize the ascending branch to the upper lobe or posterior segmental artery and, if accessible, ligate and divide. This branch may come from the dorsal segmental artery, or may be better viewed when the upper lobe bronchus has been cleaned.

(5) At this stage the fissure can be completed between upper and lower lobes, either by dissection or with the stapler.

(6) Retract the lung forward. From the rear free upper lobe bronchus, including the lymph node in the carina, between upper and intermediate bronchi. Pick up the large artery alongside the bronchus, then staple the bronchus to complete the lobectomy.

Right middle lobectomy

(1) From the lateral aspect expose and dissect the oblique fissure between middle and lower lobe.

(2) Remove lymph node at the back of the middle lobe to expose interlobar pulmonary artery.

(3) Find the dorsal segmental artery and the middle lobar artery at about the same level. There may be several middle lobe arteries. Ligate and divide these to expose the bronchus to the middle lobe medial to the junction of middle lobe artery and basal artery; divide this and close.

(4) Go to the front. Clean the anterior hilus to the inferior pulmonary vein.

(5) On examining superior pulmonary vein, middle lobe veins can be identified, ligated and divided.

(6) Complete the fissure, being wary of the interlobar pulmonary artery and its upper and lower lobe branches.

Right lower lobectomy

(1) Lateral approach: identify interlobar portion of the pulmonary artery, in front of the oblique and horizontal fissure junction and behind the middle lobe lymph gland, which can be carefully removed.
(2) See, ligate and divide dorsal segmental artery (NB there may be two of these, or superior segmental branch supplying posterior segment of right upper lobe).
(3) Ligate and divide pulmonary artery.
(4) Go to below lung, mobilize the ligament, find inferior pulmonary vein. Ligate or staple and divide. The bronchus to the lower lobe is now visible.
(5) Identify dorsal segment bronchus and ligate distally, suture proximally and divide. A few patients may have two bronchi to this segment. Then staple the basal bronchus and divide.

Right pneumonectomy

(1) Clean the pleural reflection all round the hilum, just behind the phrenic nerve, the front over the superior surface, just below the azygos vein and down the posterior surface, just anterior to the oesophagus. From the front clean right pulmonary artery, clamp, divide and suture.
(2) If shortened pulmonary artery, open pericardium, mobilize superior vena cava and take pulmonary artery lateral to the ascending aorta behind the superior vena cava. This is also a useful pressure point if the pulmonary artery is breached at other times.
(3) Superior pulmonary vein is easily freed anteriorly, superiorly and inferiorly, but posteriorly there is a dense fibrous reflection of the pericardium which should be dissected off under direct vision.
(4) Encircle the vein with a finger and ligate or staple and divide. Then the inferior pulmonary vein, which is behind and below the other structures, should be similarly divided. These veins can be divided intrapericardially and if tumour extends that far, that portion of phrenic nerve may, if necessary, also be sacrificed.
(5) If necessary, a portion of left atrial wall may be removed, but beware the orifices of veins of the opposite lung.

(6) From behind, clean nodes of the exposed carina and 1 cm of right main bronchus.
(7) Visualize left main bronchus clearly.
(8) Get the one or two bronchial arteries on the posterior surface of the main bronchus, then apply stapler as close to the carina as possible, divide and remove.

Left upper lobectomy

(1) Clean pleura from pulmonary ligament, over the front of the hilus and down the back between the vagus nerve and the lung.
(2) Expose lateral surface of pulmonary artery from the top of the hilus through into lobar fissure, being aware that a superior hilar vein may be immediately superficial to the pulmonary artery and should be ligated and divided before starting on the branch division.
(3) Clean the artery and visualize the left recurrent nerve and the ligamentum arteriosum.
(4) Dissect anterior segmental artery and apical, which may be together, but a lymph node is always between them, frequently calcified and the artery may crack as the hard lymph node presses upon it. Beware also the lingular artery coming off at this high level and passing anterior to the bronchus. This can be seen by retracting the apical posterior vein with the superior pulmonary vein.
(5) Divide the posterior and anterior segmental vessels, being aware that sometimes the dorsal segmental artery may come off the posterior segmental artery of the upper lobe.
(6) Normally the lingular vessels come off distal to the dorsal segmental artery. The lingular vessels are single in half the patients. Ligate and divide them.
(7) From the front see superior pulmonary vein. (NB about one-fifth of patients have a vein from lingula to anterior basal segment of lower lobe).
(8) The superior pulmonary vein is easily dissected inferiorly, anteriorly and superiorly, but behind there is a dense fascial layer connecting it to the bronchus. This must be divided by sharp dissection. Ligate and divide this vein, clean lymph nodes and fascia around upper lobe bronchus, then staple and divide it.

Left lower lobectomy

(1) Divide pleura over hilum, beginning at the bottom of pulmonary ligament, go up around the back in front of the oesophagus,

avoiding direct coagulation of it. Beware sequestration arteries coming in pulmonary ligament. Beware phrenic nerve as the anterior hilar cleaning is done. Confirm that there is both a superior and inferior pulmonary vein.

(2) Lateral aspect into fissure, perhaps having to divide fusion between lingula and lower lobe; with the thumb in the fissure and a finger behind the hilum, pulmonary artery may be palpated and thus exposed. Clean its lateral surface.

(3) Identify artery to dorsal segment, which comes off above the level of the lingula. Divide after ligation, after ensuring that the posterior segmental artery of the upper lobe is not coming off the dorsal segmental artery, or that the dorsal segmental artery is not arising from the apico-anterior or posterior arteries of the upper lobe.

(4) Identify and spare lingular arteries. Ligate basal segmental arteries.

(5) Complete fissure between upper and lower lobes, confirming that the inferior lingular vein does not empty into the inferior pulmonary vein.

(6) Lift lung up to expose inferior aspect, isolate inferior pulmonary vein. Remember anterior, superior and inferior aspects are in loose areolar tissues, but posteriorly there is often denser tissue.

(7) Ligate, or staple and divide this vein. Be prepared to open the pericardium to divide the vein within it if tumour is too near.

(8) Move back to front of fissure, clean lower lobe bronchi. Beware excessive traction on lower lobe bronchus, drawing upper lobe bronchus down to simulate an intermediate bronchus of which there is none in the left side.

(9) Define the dorsal segmental bronchus, confirm it arises from beyond the upper lobe bronchi and, if so, staple the lower lobe bronchus and divide.

Left pneumonectomy

(1) Clean around the pleural reflection from inferior edge of pulmonary ligament, along anterior aspect posterior to phrenic nerve, over superior border below the arch of the aorta and down the posterior aspect, anterior to descending aorta and oesophagus.

(2) Postero-superiorly free pulmonary artery, clearing the lymph nodes from under the arch of the aorta superior to it, identifying recurrent laryngeal and ligamentum arteriosum. Beware cautery near recurrent nerve of the blood vessels to the lymphatics in this area.

(3) If necessary, divide ligamentum arteriosum to get enough pulmonary artery, but do not go beyond the bifurcation of the pulmonary artery with the clamp. Dissect around the pulmonary artery with a finger and preferably clamp and oversew or staple and divide the vessel.

(4) Move to front and define superior pulmonary vein, pass a finger round it, ligate or staple and divide.

(5) Move down to inferior pulmonary vein, best done from posterior aspect, ligate or staple and divide.

(6) From posterior aspect also clean lymph nodes under carina and along opposite main bronchus.

(7) Carefully identify, ligate and divide the left bronchial arteries. NB. Two may arise direct from the aorta; these may be ligated or ligaclipped.

(8) The left main bronchus can be free for 2 cm and closed with a row of staples adjacent to the carina, the bronchus divided and the lung removed.

Complications following pulmonary resection

Post-pneumonectomy space

Management of drains is directed at maintaining trachea central and expanding all remaining lung. Bleeding over 200 ml/h for four consecutive hours or more than 500 ml in any hour are indications for re-opening.

Mediastinal shift of a massive degree and cardiac prolapse can cause a picture very like a massive pulmonary embolism or myocardial infarction. Mediastinal shift from unwise suction on the tube can quickly be corrected by releasing drain to air. A cardiac prolapse must be treated by exploration and the return of the heart to the pericardial sac past the neck which has been strangulating it. The pericardium should then be made sufficiently competent to contain the heart reliably, or opened fully,

Bronchopleural fistula

After pulmonary resection, bronchopleural fistula may be suspected if the patient develops abundant serosanguinous sputum, purulent discharge from thoracotomy wound and changes in the chest X-ray fluid level.

Early bronchopleural fistula is probably the result of failure of technique and should be repaired using direct resuturing or additional extrapleural or transpericardial closure with or without small muscle flaps.

Late bronchopleural fistula merits closed drainage to avoid mediastinal shift or open drainage with rib resection.

The bronchial stump may be cauterized using acetic acid and sodium hydroxide though periodic bronchoscopies. Also, fibrin glue or pedicled muscle flaps can be used.

Lung transplantation

The main indications for single lung transplantation are end stage pulmonary fibrosis (not expected to survive more than 12 months) in a patient aged 20–55 years, off steroids, with adequate cardiac function, no active sepsis or organ failure and psychosocial stability.

Pre-operative assessment includes lung function tests, echocardiography, lung biopsy, immunological profile, angiography, pulmonary pressures, psychiatric evaluation and full nutritional assessment.

The donors must be under 35 years with proved brain death, absence of heart or lung disease, chest X-rays with no infiltrates, good blood gases and low inflation pressure.

Immunosuppression is achieved by cyclosporin and methylprednisolone pre-operatively and with cyclosporin, azathioprine and antithymocytic globulin postoperatively.

Clinical rejection is detected by high temperature, elevated white blood cell count, hypoxaemia, abnormal chest X-ray and nuclear scans, bronchoalveolar lavage and biopsy.

The advantages of single lung transplant are:

(a) no cardiopulmonary bypass is necessary;
(b) there will be another lung available for a different patient;
(c) the cough reflex will be maintained.

The main contraindications are:

(a) pulmonary sepsis;
(b) emphysema (the ventilation will go to the diseased lung, the blood to the transplanted one and mediastinal shift may occur);
(c) right ventricular failure.

Alternatives to single lung transplant are:

(1) *Heart-lung transplant*. It has the advantage of removal of all diseased tissue, presence of airway anastomosis in the mediastinum, feasibility of rejection diagnosis by endomyocardial bi-

opsy and better tracheal vascularization. The indications for heart-lung transplant are: pulmonary vascular disease, emphysema, pulmonary sepsis and pulmonary fibrosis.

(2) *Double lung transplant*, useful in cystic fibrosis, septic pulmonary disease and emphysema.

Section VI.

Oesophageal Surgery

Oesophageal investigations

Oesophagoscopy (Figure 6.1)

This may be rigid or fibreoptic, diagnostic or therapeutic.

Indications

(1) Diagnostic: dysphagia, reflux oesophagitis, investigation of tumours.
(2) Therapeutic: resection of pediculated small tumours, dilatation with bougies, extraction of foreign bodies, and insertion of tubes through carcinomatous oesophagi.

Care should be taken with rigid instruments if an aortic aneurysm or spinal deformities are present. The main complication of the procedure is perforation; the cervical constriction, the bronchoaortic constriction and the diaphragmatic constriction are the narrow

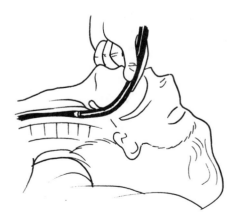

Figure 6.1 Introducing the oesophagoscope

156

points liable to perforation. The commonest cause of perforation, however, is dilatation of a stricture.

Oesophageal pressures

Using perfused catheters with side holes, or electronic probes with microtransducers, the upper sphincter pressure is found to be 70–180 mmHg and the lower sphincter pressure 15–30 mmHg.

Oesophageal pH

This is normally 5–7. Provocation of the reflux of gastric acid may change this.

Acid perfusion reveals inflamed hypersensitive lower gullet (Bernstein test).

Prolonged pH recording may show frequency on duration of reflux episodes over the course of an average day.

Reflux may be:
0: None.
1: Few episodes with normal clearance.
2: Frequent episodes with normal clearance.
3: Many episodes or during sleep; delayed clearance.
4: Reflux most of the time.

Oesophageal perforation and rupture

Causes

(1) *Iatrogenic*: endoscopy, dilatations, intubations and operations.
(2) *Non-iatrogenic*: spontaneous, foreign body, thoracic trauma, tumour, infections and burns.

Incidence

Iatrogenic: 58%; spontaneous: 19%; trauma: 16%; foreign body: 7%.

Clinical findings

Fever, mediastinal emphysema, pyrexia. Dionosil swallow confirms a leakage.

Treatment

Minor iatrogenic leaks in a well prepared patient not associated with severe pain or lack of well-being may be treated by pharyngeal and gastric intubation and suction, plus intravenous feeding for 5–6 days following carefully and closely the patient's condition.

Surgical approach may be:

- direct suture and reinforcement with pleural, gastric, intercostal or diaphragmatic patch
- exclusion and diversion in continuity
- exclusion and total diversion with cervical oesophagostomy
- gastrostomy and oesophageal ligature
- local resection and anastomosis
- resection and total diversion
- T-tube drainage.

Oesophageal carcinoma

Incidence

Upper third: 15%
Middle third: 52%
Lower third: 33%

Adenocarcinoma is more common in the lower third, probably arising in gastric mucosa. Above this, squamous tumours are more common.

TNM classification

TSM	Tumour in mucosa or submucosa
TMP	Tumour in the muscular propria
TA1	Tumour limited by the adventitia
TA2	Tumour into the adventitia
TA3	Tumour in nearby structures
N0	No metastatic node
N1	Tumour in para-oesophageal nodes of the involved segment
N3	Tumour in para-oesophageal nodes of distant oesophagus
N4	Tumour in distant nodes
M0	No distant metastases
M1	Distant metastases

Advanced disease is suggested by supraclavicular nodes, hoarseness, enlarged axillary nodes, thyroid enlargement, fixation of larynx, cough, or lung and bone metastases.

Treatment

The philosophy is to resect if physically possible (in contrast to lung, where resection is for prognostic reasons, here resection is for palliative and symptomatic reasons).
The middle and lower third are most amenable to resection. Intubation is a very poor substitute and may hasten death.
Anastomosis of the gullet above the tumour to stomach or a jejunal loop may yield superior palliation.

Oesophageal resection (left thoracotomy)

(1) Left thoracotomy above seventh rib, all the way to the costochondral junction.
(2) Tape gullet above and below tumour and mobilize tumour.
(3) Incise diaphragm circumferentially and incise all round the hiatus with finger in the abdomen to guide the hiatal circumcision.
(4) Mobilize greater curve of the stomach, gastroepiploic and short gastric arteries.
(5) Divide lesser omentum.
(6) Draw cardia through hiatus and then the stomach through hiatus.
(7) Locate left gastric artery, now above the diaphragm, and ligate/divide only if necessary.
(8) Divide oesophagogastric junction having stapled it.
(9) Bring greater curve to oesophagus at upper end, introducing stapler base through small gastrostomy.
(10) Put anvil onto stapler and divide oesophagus and pass purse string through it, using the special clamp.
(11) Introduce the anvil into the upper oesophagus, tie the purse string and close, fire and remove stapler.
(12) Finger in stapler gastrostomy to confirm perfection of anastomosis and at the same time confirm that the tissue doughnuts on the stapler are complete. With the finger in the stomach guide sump type nasogastric tube through the pylorus.
(13) Close gastrostomy, drain and close wound.

Postoperatively the main problem is bronchopneumonia which can almost invariably be prevented by avoidance of gastrobronchial overspill. Therefore the stomach must be scrupulously empty with the sump drain 'sumping' at all times.

The patient must be kept upright for the rest of his life, and when the anastomosis is confirmed sound by Gastrografin swallow at one week, metoclopramide is started in full dosage before removing the sump tube and starting oral feeding.

Appendix A

Conversion of stones and pounds into kilograms (kg)

Stones	0	1	2	3	4	5	6 (lbs)	7	8	9	10	11	12	13
0		0.5	0.9	1.4	1.8	2.3	2.7	3.2	3.6	4.1	4.5	5.0	5.4	5.9
1	6.4	6.8	7.3	7.7	8.2	8.6	9.1	9.5	10.0	10.4	10.9	11.3	11.8	12.2
2	12.7	13.2	13.6	14.1	14.5	15.0	15.4	15.9	16.3	16.8	17.2	17.7	18.1	18.6
3	19.1	19.5	20.0	20.4	20.9	21.3	21.8	22.2	22.7	23.1	23.6	24.0	24.5	24.9
4	25.4	25.9	26.3	26.8	27.2	27.7	28.1	28.6	29.0	29.5	29.9	30.4	30.8	31.3
5	31.8	32.2	32.7	33.1	33.6	34.0	34.5	34.9	35.4	35.8	36.3	36.7	37.2	37.6
6	38.1	38.6	39.0	39.5	39.9	40.4	40.8	41.3	41.7	42.2	42.6	43.1	43.5	44.0
7	44.5	44.9	45.4	45.8	46.3	46.7	47.2	47.6	48.1	48.5	49.0	49.4	49.9	50.3
8	50.8	51.3	51.7	52.2	52.6	53.1	53.5	54.0	54.4	54.9	55.3	55.8	56.2	56.7
9	57.2	57.6	58.1	58.5	59.0	59.4	59.9	60.3	60.8	61.2	61.7	62.1	62.6	63.0
10	63.5	64.0	64.4	64.9	65.3	65.8	66.2	66.7	67.1	67.6	68.0	68.5	68.9	69.4
11	69.9	70.3	70.8	71.2	71.7	72.1	72.6	73.0	73.5	73.9	74.4	74.8	75.3	75.7
12	76.2	76.7	77.1	77.6	78.0	78.5	78.9	79.4	79.8	80.3	80.7	81.2	81.6	82.1
13	82.6	83.0	83.5	83.9	84.4	84.8	85.3	85.7	86.2	86.6	87.1	87.5	88.0	88.5
14	88.9	89.4	89.8	90.3	90.7	91.2	91.6	92.1	92.5	93.0	93.4	93.9	94.3	94.8
15	95.3	95.7	96.2	96.6	97.1	97.5	98.0	98.4	98.9	99.3	99.8	100.2	100.7	101.2
16	101.6	102.1	102.5	103.0	103.4	103.9	104.3	104.8	105.2	105.7	106.1	106.6	107.0	107.5
17	108.0	108.4	108.9	109.3	109.8	110.2	110.7	111.1	111.6	112.0	112.5	112.9	113.4	113.9
18	114.3	114.8	115.2	115.7	116.1	116.6	117.0	117.5	117.9	118.4	118.8	119.3	119.7	120.2
19	120.7	121.1	121.6	122.0	122.5	122.9	123.4	123.8	124.3	124.7	125.2	125.6	126.1	126.6
20	127.0													

Appendix B

Table of average heights/weights

Men				Women			
Height	*Weight*			*Height*	*Weight*		
5′ 3″	9 st	8 lb	60.9 kg	4′ 11″	8 st	3 lb	52.3 kg
5′ 4″	9 st	10 lb	61.8 kg	5′	8 st	5 lb	53.2 kg
5′ 5″	10 st	1 lb	64.1 kg	5′ 1″	8 st	7 lb	54.1 kg
5′ 6″	10 st	4 lb	65.5 kg	5′ 2″	8 st	9 lb	55.0 kg
5′ 7″	10 st	8 lb	67.3 kg	5′ 3″	8 st	12 lb	56.4 kg
5′ 8″	10 st	11 lb	68.5 kg	5′ 4″	9 st	1 lb	57.7 kg
5′ 9″	11 st	2 lb	70.9 kg	5′ 5″	9 st	5 lb	59.5 kg
5′ 10″	11 st	6 lb	72.7 kg	5′ 6″	9 st	8 lb	60.9 kg
5′ 11″	11 st	11 lb	75.0 kg	5′ 7″	9 st	12 lb	62.7 kg
6′	12 st	2 lb	77.3 kg	5′ 8″	10 st	2 lb	64.5 kg
6′ 1″	12 st	7 lb	79.5 kg	5′ 9″	10 st	6 lb	66.3 kg
6′ 2″	12 st	11 lb	81.4 kg	5′ 10″	10 st	10 lb	68.2 kg
6′ 3″	13 st	1 lb	83.2 kg	5′ 11″	11 st	0 lb	70.0 kg
				6′	11 st	4 lb	71.8 kg

Appendix C

Conversion of feet and inches to centimetres (cm)

NB. This table scans vertically, not in the normal horizontal manner.

Inches	0	1	2	Feet 3	4	5	6
0	–	30.5	61.0	91.4	121.9	152.4	182.9
½	1.3	31.8	62.2	92.7	123.2	153.7	184.2
1	2.5	33.0	63.5	94.0	124.5	154.9	185.4
1½	3.8	34.3	64.8	95.3	125.7	156.2	186.7
2	5.1	35.6	66.0	96.5	127.0	157.5	188.0
2½	6.4	36.8	67.3	97.8	128.3	158.8	189.2
3	7.6	38.1	68.6	99.1	129.5	160.0	190.5
3½	8.9	39.4	69.9	100.3	130.8	161.3	191.8
4	10.2	40.6	71.1	101.6	132.1	162.6	193.0
4½	11.4	41.9	72.4	102.9	133.4	163.8	194.3
5	12.7	43.2	73.7	104.1	134.6	165.1	195.6
5½	14.0	44.5	74.9	105.4	135.9	166.4	196.9
6	15.2	45.7	76.2	106.7	137.2	167.6	198.1
6½	16.5	47.0	77.5	108.0	138.4	168.9	199.4
7	17.8	48.3	78.7	109.2	139.7	170.2	200.7
7½	19.1	49.5	80.0	110.5	141.0	171.5	201.9
8	20.3	50.8	81.3	111.8	142.2	172.7	203.2
8½	21.6	52.1	82.6	113.0	143.5	174.0	204.5
9	22.9	53.3	83.8	114.3	144.8	175.3	205.7
9½	24.1	54.6	85.1	115.6	146.1	176.5	207.0
10	25.4	55.9	86.4	116.8	147.3	177.8	208.3
10½	26.7	57.2	87.6	118.1	148.6	179.1	209.6
11	27.9	58.4	88.9	119.4	149.9	180.3	210.8
11½	29.2	59.7	90.2	120.7	151.1	181.6	212.1

Appendix D

Conversion of degrees Fahrenheit to degrees Celsius

Body temperatures

°F	°C	°F	°C
86	30	98	36.7
86.5	30.3	98.4	36.9
87	30.6	99	37.2
87.5	30.8	99.5	37.5
88	31.1	100	37.8
88.5	31.4	100.4	38.0
89	31.7	101	38.3
89.5	31.9	101.5	38.6
90	32.2	102	38.9
90.5	32.5	102.5	39.2
91	32.8	103	39.4
91.5	33.1	103.5	39.7
92	33.3	104	40.0
92.5	33.6	104.5	40.3
93	33.9	105	40.6
93.5	34.2	105.5	40.8
94	34.4	106	41.1
94.5	34.7	106.5	41.4
95	35	107	41.7
95.5	35.3	107.5	41.9
96	35.6	108	42.2
96.5	35.8	108.5	42.5
97	36.1	109	42.8
97.5	36.4	109.5	43.1

Other temperatures in common use:

32 °F	=	0 °C	120 °F	approx.	49 °C
60 °F	approx.	16 °C	160 °F	approx.	71 °C
70 °F	approx.	21 °C	180 °F	approx.	82 °C
80 °F	approx.	27 °C	212 °F	=	100 °C
110 °F	approx.	43 °C	250 °F	approx.	121 °C
115 °F	approx.	46 °C	259 °F	approx.	126 °C
			273 °F	approx.	134 °C

Appendix E

Dilution table

1% 10 ml diluted to 1000 ml (1 in 100)
0.1% 1 ml diluted to 1000 ml (1 in 1000)
0.01% 0.1 ml diluted to 1000 ml (1 in 10000)

Further Reading

Section I. Cardiac Medicine

Shock

SHINE, K. *et al.* (1980). Aspects of the management of shock. *Annals of Internal Medicine*, **93**, 723

Cardiorespiratory arrest

ROSEQUIST, C. (1987). Current standards and guidelines for cardiopulmonary resuscitation and emergency cardiac care. *Heart and Lung*, **16**, 408

Cardiac arrhythmias

ARNSDORF, M. (1984). Basic understanding of the electrophysiologic actions of antiarrhythmic drugs: sources, sinks and matrices of information. *Medical Clinics of North America*, **68**, 1247

Anti-arrhythmic drugs

CAMPBELL, R. W. F. (Ed.) (1987). Clinical usefulness of antiarrhythmic drugs. *European Heart Journal*, **8** (Suppl. A), 1–137

Pacemakers

HARTHORNE, J. (1981). Indications for pacemaker insertion: types and mode of pacing. *Progress in Cardiovascular Diseases*, **23**, 393–400
ZAIDAN, J. (1984). Pacemakers. *Anesthesiology*, **60**, 319–334

Heart failure

HERMANOVICH, J. (1985). Management of cardiac patient requiring non-cardiac surgery. *Surgical Clinics of North America*, **63**, 985
HILLIS, W. and BEEN, M. (1984). Cardiac failure. In *Cardiovascular Update* (ed. G. Jackson), Update Publications, London, pp. 63–70.

165

Inotropics used in heart failure

FOEX, P. (1983). Inotropics and vasodilator agents. In *Recent Advances in Critical Care Medicine, 2*, Churchill Livingstone, London.

Acute pulmonary oedema

STAUB, N. (1980). The pathogenesis of pulmonary oedema. *Progress in Cardiovascular Disease*, **23**, 53

Ischaemic heart disease

FALK, E. (1985). Unstable angina with fatal outcome: dynamic coronary thrombosis leading to infarction and sudden death. *Circulation*, **71**, 699

LEAMAN, D. and DAVIS, O. (1983). Diagnosis and management of myocardial ischemia in the postoperative period. *Surgical Clinics of North America*, **63**, 1081

Myocardial infarction

STARLING, R., WALKER, W., WERLAND, A. *et al*. (1984). Early bypass grafting following intracoronary thrombolysis with streptokinase. *Journal of Thoracic and Cardiovascular Surgery*, **87**, 487

Complicated myocardial infarction

BOURKE, J. and COWAN, C. (1986). Ventricular arrhythmias after myocardial infarction. *Current Opinions in Cardiology*, **1**, 483–491

COHEN, M., PARKER, M. and GORLIN, R. (1983). Indications for left ventricular aneurysmectomy. *Circulation*, **67**, 717

JATENE, A. (1985). Left ventricular aneurysmectomy. *Journal of Thoracic and Cardiovascular Surgery*, **89**, 321

KILLEN, D. *et al*. (1983). Surgical treatment of papillary muscle rupture. *Annals of Thoracic Surgery*, **35**, 243

TADAOMI, A. *et al*. (1983). Postmyocardial infarction ventricular septal defect. *Journal of Thoracic and Cardiovascular Surgery*, **86**, 41

Section II. Cardiac Surgery

Monitoring

GEORGE, R. (1985). The chemical value of measuring cardiac output. *British Journal of Hospital Medicine*, **34**, 89–95

HILL, D. and DOLAN, A. (1976). *Intensive Care Instrumentation*, Academic Press, London

SCHROEDER, J. and DAILY, E. (1976). *Techniques in Bedside Hemodynamic Monitoring*, C. V. Mosby, St Louis

Complications after coronary surgery

LOOP, F., LITTLE, B., GILL, C. *et al.* (1983). Trends in selection and results of coronary artery reoperations. *Annals of Thoracic Surgery*, **36**, 380

Valve surgery

CARPENTIER, A. (1983). Cardiac valve surgery: the French correction. *Journal of Thoracic and Cardiovascular Surgery*, **86**, 323

Infective endocarditis

KRAYENBUHL, H. and RICKARDS (Eds) (1984). New aspects of bacterial endocarditis. *European Heart Journal*, **5**, (Suppl. C), 1–146
MASUR, H. AND JOHNSON, W. (1980). Prosthetic valve endocarditis. *Journal of Thoracic and Cardiovascular Surgery*, **80**, 31

Aortic aneurysms

CARLSON, D., KARP, R. and KOUCHOUKOS, N. (1983). Surgical treatment of aneurysms of the descending aorta: an analysis of 85 patients. *Annals of Thoracic Surgery*, **35**, 5
KOUCHOUKOS, N., KARP, R., BLACKSTONE, E. *et al.* (1980). Replacement of the ascending aorta and aortic graft with a composite graft: results in 86 patients. *Annals of Surgery*, **192**, 403

Section III. Congenital Heart Disease

Cardiac arrest in children

BRAY, R. (1985). The management of cardiac arrest in infants and children. *British Journal of Hospital Medicine*, **34**, 72–81
BRAY, R. (1987). Paediatric resuscitation. *Hospital Update*, **13**, 265–278

The child with congenital heart disease

COHN, L., DOTY, D. and MCELVEIN, R. (1987). *Decision Making in Cardiothoracic Surgery*, B. C. Decker

Coarctation of the aorta

HARLAN, J., DOTY, D., BRANDT, B. and EHRENHAFT, J. (1984). Coarctation of the aorta in infants. *Journal of Thoracic and Cardiovascular Surgery*, **88**, 1012
HOLDEN, M. (1982). *A Practice of Cardiothoracic Surgery*, J. Wright, Bristol

Total anomalous pulmonary venous drainage

HAWKINS, J., CLARK, E. and DOTY, B. (1983). Total anomalous pulmonary venous connection. *Annals of Thoracic Surgery* **36**, 548

Section IV. Respiratory Medicine

Respiratory failure

FLENLEY, D. (1981). *Respiratory Medicine*, Bailliere-Tindall, London

Adult respiratory distress syndrome

SHALE, D. (1987). The adult respiratory distress syndrome. *Thorax*, **42**, 641

Mechanical ventilation

MORTIMER, A. and SYKES, M. (1983). Monitoring of ventilation. In *Recent Advances in Critical Care Medicine*, **2**, Churchill Livingstone, London

Pulmonary embolism

GLASSFORS, D., ALFORD, W., BURRUS, G. *et al.* (1981). Pulmonary embolectomy. *Annals of Thoracic Surgery*, **32**, 28

HALL, R. (1985). Difficulties in the treatment of acute pulmonary embolism. *Thorax*, **40**, 729

STEIN, P., WILLIS, P. and DALEN, J. (1979). Importance of clinical assessment in selecting patient for pulmonary arteriography. *American Journal of Cardiology*, **43**, 669

Massive haemoptysis

CONLAN, A., HURWITZ, S., KRIGE, L. and POOLE, R. (1983). Massive haemoptysis. *Journal of Thoracic and Cardiovascular Surgery*, **85**, 120

MARGOLES, J. (1963). Balloon tamponade for massive pulmonary hemorrhage. *Annals of Surgery*, **86**, 83

Pneumonia

STRATTON, A. (1986). Bacterial pneumonias: an overview with emphasis on pathogenesis, diagnosis and treatment. *Heart-Lung*, **15**, 226

Acute emergencies in asthma

PATERSON, J., WOOLCOCK, A. and SHENFIELD, G. (1979). Bronchodilator drugs. *American Review of Respiratory Diseases*, **120**, 1149–1188

Section V. Thoracic Surgery

Cardiothoracic trauma

CONN, J., HARDY, J., FAIN, W. *et al.* (1963). Thoracic trauma: analysis of 1022 cases. *Journal of Trauma*, **3**, 22

HARLEY, D., MENA, I., MIRANDA, R. *et al.* (1983). Myocardial contusion following blunt trauma. *Archives of Surgery*, **118**, 1384

RICHARDSON, J., MCELVEIN, R. and TRINKLE, J. (1975). First rib fracture: a hallmark of severe trauma. *Annals of Surgery*, **181**, 251

Lung abscess

LE ROUX, B. *et al.* (1986). Suppurative diseases of the lung and pleural space. Part I: Empyema thoracis and lung abscess. *Current Problems in Surgery*, **23**, 38

Septic shock

WILES, J. *et al.* (1980). The systemic septic response: does the organism matter? *Critical Care Medicine*, **8**, 55

Multisystem failure in surgical patients

HENAO, F. and ALDRETE, J. (1985). Multiple systems organ failure: is it a specific entity? *Southern Medical Journal*, **78**, 329

Foreign bodies in airways

CHATTERGI, S. and CHATTERGI, P. (1972). The management of foregn bodies in air passages. *Anaesthesia*, **27**, 390

EDITORIAL (1972). Drowning. *Lancet*, **ii**, 69

HARRISON, M. (1972). Inhaled foreign body. *Anaesthesia*, **27**, 478

Lung cancer

CHUNG, C. *et al.* (1982). Carcinoma of the lung: evaluation of histological grade and factors affecting prognosis. *Annals of Thoracic Surgery*, **33**, 599

Lung transplantation

KAMHOLZ, S. *et al.* (1983). Single lung transplantation with cyclosporin immunosuppression. *Journal of Thoracic and Cardiovascular Surgery*, **86**, 537

Index